Primer on Measurement: An Introductory Guide to Measurement Issues

Featuring the American Physical Therapy Association's
Standards for Tests and Measurements in Physical Therapy Practice

Jules M Rothstein, PhD, PT, FAPTA
Professor and Head, Department of Physical Therapy (M/C 898)
University of Illinois at Chicago, and
Chief of Physical Therapy Services
University of Illinois Hospital, 1919 W Taylor St, Chicago, IL 60612 (USA)

John L Echternach, EdD, PT, FAPTA
Eminent Professor
School of Community Health Professions and Physical Therapy
Old Dominion University, Norfolk, VA 23539-0288 (USA)

Contents

Acknowledgments

The *Standards for Tests and Measurements in Physical Therapy Practice* were generated by the American Physical Therapy Association's Task Force on Standards for Measurement in Physical Therapy. Two members of that group authored the *Primer*. The authors are grateful to their colleagues on the Task Force—Suzann K Campbell, PhD, PT, FAPTA, Alan M Jette, PhD, PT, and Harry G Knecht, EdD, PT—for all their assistance in the refinement of ideas and in the preparation of this document. In addition, Anthony Delitto, PhD, PT, and Dan L Riddle, PT, provided invaluable insights in the preparation of the *Primer*. The authors especially thank Eugene Michels, PT, FAPTA, for his guidance on aspects of the project and for his development of the initial drafts and organization of this *Primer*.

Primer on Measurement: An Introductory Guide to Measurement Issues

Introduction

In August of 1991, the *Standards for Tests and Measurements in Physical Therapy Practice** were published in the journal *Physical Therapy*. That document was meant to serve as a rule book guiding clinicians in their use of tests and measurements. Rule books are supposed to be definitive and to the point; rarely are they user-friendly or easy to read. The *Standards* are no exception. One can hardly imagine anyone reading or understanding a baseball or football rule book unless that person already has some understanding of those sports. In view of the paucity of training most physical therapists have had in measurement sciences, how can they hope to understand and use the *Standards*? The *Standards*, after all, were meant to be all-inclusive and to serve as a reference—and who can easily read a reference book? The authors of the *Standards* knew that they needed a companion volume. The *Primer on Measurement* was born out of this need.

This *Primer* introduces readers to measurement issues and prepares them to use and understand the *Standards*. If you understand measurement issues, terms, and related mathematical and statistical concepts, you need not read the *Primer*. But, if you are among the many therapists who do not feel comfortable with these topics, the *Primer* can give you a sense of the "game" before you get into the rule book. And, in the opinion of the Task Force that wrote the *Standards*, it is time that more therapists understood the rules of the game of measurement. Many therapists may feel that because they take measurements, they are already familiar with the topic, but often their training in measurement has consisted of little more than learning how to obtain measurements. There is more to measurement than obtaining numbers or classifying things—you need to understand the theoretical bases for measurement, sources of error, and how to interpret clinical information. Many therapists,

---

* In August 1987, the Research Committee of the American Physical Therapy Association (APTA) proposed the development of standards of measurements in physical therapy. In November 1987, the APTA Board of Directors appointed a Task Force on Standards for Measurement in Physical Therapy. The members of the Task Force were Jules M Rothstein, PhD, PT (coordinator), Suzann K Campbell, PhD, PT, FAPTA, John L Echternach, EdD, PT, FAPTA, Alan M Jette, PhD, PT, Harry G Knecht, EdD, PT, and the late Steven J Rose, PhD, PT, FAPTA. In 1991, the *Standards* were adopted by the APTA Board of Directors and published in *Physical Therapy*. The *Standards* are reprinted as an appendix in the *Primer*. Asterisks throughout the *Primer* refer to passages in the *Standards*.

however, feel that issues such as these are relevant only to research, not to practice. We urge these therapists to read on. We believe that the issues discussed within this volume are not esoteric topics for elitists, but rather the heart and soul of good clinical practice.

The *Primer* is designed to be used by therapists and students who have, or are acquiring, the knowledge and skills required to obtain measurements. Practical examples are therefore used throughout. Sometimes, in an attempt to make each example not only relevant but also clear to the reader, we have created fictitious examples. Implications for practice are explored whenever possible. The *Primer* has no "how-to" sections, which means it does not include descriptions of how to do any tests. The *Primer* is not a manual on how to test, nor is it meant to be a source list of approved tests and procedures. Although the *Primer* does not provide a listing of which tests and measurements are good or bad, it does provide the knowledge that will allow you—the clinician—to use the *Standards* and your professional judgment to choose the best tests and measurements.

This *Primer* is a secondary reference, an overview of issues related to the *Standards*. In addition, the reader should know that in measurement sciences, there is no universal agreement about terms and ideas. In this *Primer*, terms are used as they are used in the *Standards*.

Because the *Primer* and the *Standards* are not "how-to" books, and because they contain no lists, it is easy to ask, "Why is there a set of *Standards* at all?" Measurements are taken to provide information, but the result may be *mis*information if the quality of measurements is not ensured. *The purpose of the* Standards *is to provide guidelines that will help ensure the quality of measurements.* The *Standards* are tools for practitioners, tools intended to demonstrate to society the commitment of physical therapists to practice in a credible and scientific manner. The *Standards* reflect our profession's humanistic commitment to provide the highest quality of care to our patients. The *Standards* are primarily practice-oriented but, to be all-inclusive, include sections on research and teaching. The *Standards* describe how measurements should be used in clinical practice. Through the use of the *Standards*, therapists can, in their practice settings, deliver more effective care and document the results of examination and treatment.

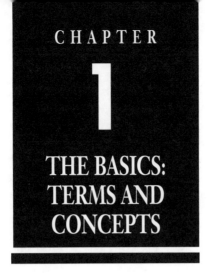

THE BASICS: TERMS AND CONCEPTS

Definitions of Terms

In the *Standards*, a **test** is defined as *"a procedure or set of procedures that is used to obtain measurements (data); the procedures may require the use of instruments."** This definition might seem distant from clinical practice, but clinicians spend a significant portion of their time obtaining measurements.

When we determine the angle to which a patient can straight leg raise, we are conducting a test (a procedure) to obtain a measurement (an angle). The process may be less obvious when we say a patient has "poor sitting balance," but here also we have engaged in the process of measurement. We have measured because we used some rule to classify the sitting ability of the patient. We sometimes are too casual about measuring and classifying. Sometimes, we do not even know what procedures we used to obtain our measurements. For example, if you were to classify a patient as needing moderate assistance for ambulation, are you aware of what procedures (rules) guided you in assigning the patient to an assistance category? Are these the same rules and categories that guide your colleagues?

To measure means *to obtain a measurement (datum).* The result of testing and measuring is the attainment of a **measurement.** The term "measurement," although frequently used in clinical and other settings, often goes undefined and taken for granted. The simplest definition of a measurement is *"the numeral assigned to an object, event, or person or the class (category) to which an object, event, or person is assigned according to rules."** A measurement applies a label to something. That label either denotes the quantity of something or the category that something belongs to. We measure when we *quantify* by determining amounts, and we measure when we *qualify* by placing objects, persons, or characteristics into categories. If we say someone has a 4-cm-long and 2-cm-wide pressure ulcer, we are measuring length and width. If we say that a pressure ulcer shows signs of healing, we are classifying the ulcer, another form of measurement. One form of measurement is quantitative, and the other is qualitative.

In order to quantify or to categorize, there must be a set of rules that guide these procedures. The rules are contained within **operational definitions.** Operational definitions are

> *... a set of procedures that guides the process of obtaining a measurement; includes descriptions of the attribute (the person, place, thing, characteristic, and so forth) that is to be measured, the conditions under which the measurement is to be taken, and the actions that are to be taken in order to obtain the measurement.**

The term **attribute** in the definition means a *"variable; a characteristic or quality that is measured."**

The amount of motion found at the glenohumeral joint is an attribute, as is the type of cerebral palsy that a child may have. Motion is an attribute described in quantitative terms (eg, degrees are used to describe the arc of motion, whereas the type of cerebral palsy is a categorical attribute). Similarly, when patients are classified as having one of the low back derangements described by McKenzie,[2] the type of derangement is the attribute.

In physical therapy, we use many terms to describe the means we use to obtain measurements. We have already defined **test** and **measurement,** but often it is not clear how these terms relate to the more commonly used clinical term **examination.** An examination is *"a test or a group of tests used for the purpose of obtaining measurements or data."** To **assess** is to measure, because assessment means to quantify or to place a numeric value or label on something. This is in contrast to **evaluation,** another word commonly used in clinical practice but rarely defined. Although some controversy exists about the definition of evaluation, in the *Standards* and throughout this *Primer* the term is used to mean *"a judgment based on a measurement; evaluations are judgments of the value or worth of something."** Although evaluation is often used as a synonym for examination, the definitions in the *Standards* should discourage this inappropriate and confusing usage.

Taking a Measurement— Where We Begin

No measurements should be obtained unless there is an identified **attribute, characteristic, property, dimension,** or **variable** to be **categorized** or **quantified.** In other words, you should not attempt to measure something unless you know what that something is. The opening sentence in this paragraph provides the list of synonyms for "attribute."

In clinical practice, the first measurement issue therapists encounter when they deal with a patient is the determination of what to measure (what to include in an examination); that is: What attributes need to be quantified or categorized? Selecting attributes to be tested in patients requires knowledge about the clinical condition, available treatments, the quality of measurements available, and so on. Most importantly, before a measurement of an attribute can be made, the attribute must be defined.

What Is an Operational Definition?

An attribute cannot be measured unless that attribute is defined. But, if that definition does not describe the process of measurement, the definition remains more theoretical than practical. Measurement requires theoretical and practical considerations. A definition that guides the process of measurement is an **operational definition,** a definition that makes evident what an attribute is and how it is measured. Defining an attribute operationally means describing what to look at (or what to look for), what to do, and how to do what is to be done in order to obtain the desired measurements.

Some of the attributes that physical therapists measure are so commonly discussed and taken for granted that we do not even realize that operational definitions exist. For example, consider the measurement of range of motion (ROM) with a goniometer. Physical therapists are trained early in entry-level education to know the various planes of motion possible at all joints of the extremities, to know the approximate normal ROMs possible at these joints, to passively move the segments of the extremities through the various planes and ROMs, to estimate the ROM possible in each plane for each joint, and to apply a goniometer to measure the ROM in each plane. Physical therapists are socialized in what to look at (or what to look for), what to do, and how to do what is to be done in order to measure the ROM of most joints with a goniometer. Someplace along the line we developed within ourselves a set of operational definitions for the measurement of motion of most joints. Ideally, a manual was used that contained operational definitions that had been tested by research. Although such manuals exist, to date none have really been validated through research.

If the socialization process (instruction) related to measurement of ROM is not accompanied by a manual, then an unwritten operational definition is formed. Does this, however, make the process of measuring joint ROM apparent? Perhaps it can be argued that instructors made ROM measurement apparent to successive classes of students by teaching them what to look at, what to do, and how to do it. But do we really know that instructors did this in a consistent fashion? And, do we know whether there is consistency among schools and regions? In addition, did we all receive similar training when it came to measurement of motion at the subtalar joint, the joints of the hand, or the spinal joints? More importantly, do we know whether there is evidence that the techniques we are using yield useful (ie, valid) information?

All too often, measurements used by physical therapists are defined implicitly rather than explicitly. For the measurement of motion at most joints, the procedures may seem apparent, and there are even manuals that describe these procedures (even though the manuals often lack scientific justification). But are there explicit and commonly agreed-upon definitions and procedures for the measurement of tone, strength, segmental mobility, and balance? When operational definitions remain implicit, they are concealed from public view, and as a result we can never be sure what is being measured or what the measurement reflects. Without an operational definition for strength, how can we interpret a report about a patient's strength? Would we know, for example, whether the patient's "strength" had been measured with an isokinetic device, with a hand-held dynamometer, by determining the weight lifted, or by any of a variety of other means?

Do all therapists have common definitions for levels of sitting balance, functional independence, tone, walking ability, or coordination? Meaningful measurements cannot be obtained unless definitions are shared, and unless we are able to understand what each therapist has done to obtain a measurement.

If measurements taken by different therapists or even by the same therapists on different occasions differ, even though the attribute being measured has not changed, then the measurement will not be useful. Measurements should reflect the attribute being measured and not other factors. If different persons measure differently because they do not observe a common operational definition, then changes in the measurement may be a function of how the measurement was obtained rather than a function of a change in the attribute. Decisions and judgments based on measurements that fluctuate without regard to the phenomenon being measured are unlikely to be correct.

Without operational definitions, we cannot even attempt to determine whether measurements are consistent (reliable). If therapists insist on "doing their own thing" each time they measure, then their measurements become unique and uninterpretable by anyone else. Often therapists modify existing measurement procedures in an attempt to obtain better measurements. In reality, this often adds to the confusion surrounding measurements.

To be useful, an operational definition must have a sound theoretical basis, and it must also be sufficiently clear to guide people in taking measurements in a way that leads to consistency. The definition should also specify the types of measurements that are obtained. For example, when we measure our patients' back motion by measuring how far their fingers are from the floor when they bend forward, we are measuring linear distance, but when we measure back motion with a goniometer, we are measuring back motion in terms of angular displacement. The operational definition for each type of measurement should specify the type of measurement that will be obtained (eg, linear or angular measurements). This example not only emphasizes the importance of operational definitions, but it also illustrates how we may attempt to measure the same phenomenon (eg, back motion) with two different methods, and that the methods may yield entirely different kinds of measurements.

The issues related to operational definitions are vast and are derived from all elements of measurement science. In this brief introduction to operational definitions, we have introduced the need for theoretical soundness in an operational definition, which relates to **validity**, and we said a good definition leads to consistency, which relates to **reliability**. In addition, we have said the definition should describe and justify the types of measurements that are obtained, which means that **scales** and **levels of measurement** must be understood before we can fully comprehend operational definitions. We must explore all of these related issues and topics before we can achieve a full understanding of operational definitions.

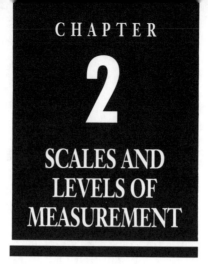

CHAPTER

2

SCALES AND LEVELS OF MEASUREMENT

Scales

Contained within an operational definition are the categories or units that will be used to characterize the attribute. Different levels of measurement may, therefore, be used to characterize attributes. For example, we categorize patients when we say that they do or do not fit into diagnostic categories, but we quantify when we measure the amount of force the quadriceps femoris muscle can generate. In each case, a different type of **scale** is used. The word scale can be defined in several ways, but the following definition provides some insight. A **scale** is

> ... *a system of ordered marks at fixed intervals used as a reference standard in measurement; a progressive classification, as of size, amount, importance, or rank.*[2]

In practice, scales consist of two or more units or categories that are **mutually exclusive** and **exhaustive**.

The term exclusive simply means that when a measurement is applied to an attribute, only one measurement would be appropriate. For example, a patient's quadriceps femoris muscle manual muscle test (MMT) grade may be F (Fair) or it may be G (Good). These grades are mutually exclusive because each grade has its own definition. If you say that a person's MMT grade was F/G, then the measurement is not exclusive unless you consider F/G as a unique grade with its own operational definition and not just a combination of grades.

The term **exhaustive** refers to the requirement that no matter what form the attribute may take, there will be a label or quantity available to describe the attribute. For example, if we were classifying patients who had cerebrovascular accidents (CVAs) and only used the categories of right or left hemiplegia, we would not have exhaustive categories. We would not have a category for persons with bilateral lesions. Our failure to be exhaustive in this case would also result in a failure to be mutually exclusive, because we would assign persons with bilateral lesions to both the right and left hemiplegic groups. In practice, there is often a category called "none of the above," "does not apply," or something similar. Although such categories provide very little information, they can be useful in preserving the legitimacy of a scale by making it exhaustive.

Sometimes, a scale may not just reflect one **(unidimensional)** element (eg, just ROM or just force production); instead, scales may be used to reflect two or more attributes at the same time. An activities-of-daily-living (ADL) scale that can be used to simultaneously measure both the relative degree of independence and the amount of time required in performing each activity is an example of a **multidimensional scale**.

The following shows how a multidimensional scale for ADL and time might be developed. We could have two categories for classifying the degree of independence:

Independent
or
Dependent

We could also have two categories for classifying the time required for a person to take care of his or her ADL needs (particularly if we knew the average time it took for most persons to perform each activity):

More Than Average (which we will call "Slow")
or
Average or Less (which we will call "Acceptable")

Now, let's look at the two ADL scales (degree of independence and time required) that we want to combine into one scale:

Variable (dimension) Categories
Independence: **Dependent**   or   **Independent**
Time Required: **Slow**   or   **Acceptable**

Simply combining the two categories on the left into one category and then the two categories on the right into one category would create a scale that consists of only two categories:

Dependent-Slow
or
Independent-Acceptable

The combination with just two categories creates an unworkable scale and an inadequate number of categories because the performance of patients who tested as **Dependent-Acceptable** and patients who tested as **Independent-Slow** would not fit into any group. To satisfy the logical requirement for mutually exclusive and exhaustive categories on the combination of two scales, we would have to provide for **all possible combinations** of each category on the one scale with all categories on the other scale. This would lead to four groups:

Dependent-Slow
Dependent-Acceptable
Independent-Slow
Independent-Acceptable

Combining scales is more complex if one or more of the scales have more than two categories, and if more than two scales are combined. If two scales are combined, the resultant number of categories on the combined scale will be the product of the number of categories on the one original scale and the number of categories on the other original scale. For our example above, the number of categories on the combined scale is four (the product of 2x2). If each of the two original scales had three categories, the combined scale would have 3x3=9 categories.

If three scales are to be combined, and if each of the original three scales had three categories, the combined scale would have 3x3x3=27 categories.

Combining scales, therefore, may be desirable, but it should always be done with a theoretical basis and an appreciation of the complexity that will result from multidimensional scales.

Poor examples of multiple attributes and their combined scales can often be found among rating scales used to assess the performance of staff or the performance of students in clinical education. Some of these flawed combinations of multiple attributes are deceptive because they look simple, often requiring basic "yes" or "no" answers, and they often look attractive because they are value-laden. Items containing highly valued attributes are not likely to receive critical scrutiny. Here are two examples, each to be answered "yes" or "no," from instruments designed to test student performance:

1. Maintains confidentiality of patient's records and conversations.
2. Adjusts verbal and nonverbal communication to each person and situation.

The first example tests two attributes: maintaining confidentiality of records **and** maintaining confidentiality of conversations. A student could maintain confidentiality of records but not conversations, or vice versa. If confidentiality was not maintained for either, the answer must be "no." A person using the scale would then be unable to know which incorrect behavior the student engaged in. By combining two attributes into one question, some information is lost, but an argument can be made that by combining the two attributes, the question deals with a general issue of whether the student is able to maintain confidentiality. The two attributes should not be combined unless the persons who developed the instrument believe that by combining the attributes, they will form a single index that reflects a single underlying element (construct). If a case is made that a single construct is being measured, then there must be clear instructions as to how a Clinical Instructor is to grade the student, in other words, how the variables can be combined into a single judgment.

The second example tests four attributes: adjusting verbal communication to each person, adjusting verbal communication to each situation, adjusting nonverbal communication to each person, and adjusting nonverbal communication to each situation. One would really have to wonder what a simple "yes" or "no" answer would mean. In this second example, the combination does not provide information on a simple behavior with two variants (such as in the example about maintaining confidentiality), but rather has an unmanageable mix of elements. Because there are no instructions on how to combine the various observations to form a single judgment, multiple users of this instrument will be unlikely to make reliable judgments.

Sometimes, however, it is very useful to combine measurements of multiple attributes to form a single **index.** Clinicians often base decisions not on measurements of single variables, but rather on measurements of multiple variables. Ideally, this should be done in a systematic fashion in which the method of combination and the contribution of each variable to the final index are defined. Indices that reflect **multivariate** phenomena can be very useful in clinical practice, but they are difficult to develop and must be examined for all the qualities that make a measurement acceptable (eg, whether they are reliable and valid).

For example, is it really reasonable to expect muscle force measurements to be useful in predicting functional activities? Even persons who have total paralysis of the muscles normally used in gait can still walk, albeit with some gait deviations, but, as was often noted in persons with paralysis due to poliomyelitis, there often were no observable gait deviations.[3] Apparently, the ability to walk reflects not just force measurements from a single muscle, but rather the ability of multiple muscles to generate force and a person's skill in using these muscles in a coordinated fashion. Therefore, an index that could predict the function of walking would be needed to reflect multiple variables.

Many indices already exist, such as the Modified Oswestry Scale for Low Back Pain,[4,5] which combines elements to provide a single score that reflects the impact of low back pain. Instead of using this index, clinicians could, for example, ask a variety of questions about their patient's pain and function and attempt to make judgments based on each question or based on some unspecified interpretation of how answers related to one another. Or, they could use this scale to provide a single index (measure) to reflect the various elements in the questionnaire. Indices can provide single scores (derived measurements) that reflect complex phenomena. Some other indices used by physical therapists are the Barthel Index, which reflects ADL status,[6] and the Motor Assessment for Infants (MAI),[7,8] which is used to reflect the motor development of infants. Indices are often derived from multiple measurements (or questions) combined in a systematic manner. Later in the *Primer*, **derived measurements** are discussed. All the issues in that discussion relate to indices.

One important difference between an index and other uses of combined measurements is that with an index, there is a specified manner in which various components are combined. This allows for the development of indices that can be used in similar ways by different clinicians. The *ad hoc* combination of measurements to form indices often results in derived measurements that meet none of the criteria for acceptable measurements. Clinicians should be wary of combining measurements to form single indices unless there is evidence to suggest that the index is useful and provides meaningful information.

Levels of Measurement

Most experts in tests and measurements agree that there are four levels or scales for tests and measurements: **ratio**, **interval**, **ordinal**, and **nominal**. In this *Primer*, we accept the premise that there are four levels of measurement.

Ratio Scales

Examples of measurements based on a ratio scale in physical therapy are ROM (measured in degrees), limb length, time to complete an activity, vital capacity, and nerve conduction velocity.

A ratio scale has a zero point that represents the complete absence of the quantity represented. The intervals among all successive units on the scale must be equal in size. A measurement on a ratio scale, therefore, cannot have a minus or a negative value. For example, a person could not have a negative conduction velocity or a negative chest circumference.

Imagine a person who can move his or her leg through an arc of motion such that at one extreme (flexion) the tibia forms a 120-degree angle with the femur and at the other extreme (extension) it forms a 30-degree angle. To say the person exhibits "-30 degrees" of extension is incorrect. You cannot possibly have less than no motion! The common use of phrases such as "-30 degrees of motion" does not make this terminology acceptable or useful. When we use jargon and shortcuts to describe measurements, as in saying someone has "-30 degrees of motion," we not only disregard the level of measurement being used, we also engage in potentially confusing descriptions that interfere with communication and documentation.

Would all therapists agree as to what "-30 degrees of extension" really meant? Would we all share a common image about a patient who we were told has "-10 degrees of medial rotation at the shoulder"? Perhaps some confusion occurs because negative measurements are used to characterize deficits (often the presence of impairments). Deficits and negative measurements are not the same. A negative value may not exist if the measurement is ratio scaled. You can correctly say that a person lacks 20 degrees of knee flexion, but only if a frame of reference is specified. What value was expected that led to the conclusion that 20 degrees was lacking? In this case, there is not a negative value for the measurement, but rather a statement of what is lacking.

Because ratio-scaled measurements have a zero point representing an absence of the quantity being measured and because the intervals among successive levels of measurement are equally spaced, ratio-scaled measurements can be subjected to all arithmetic operations. The very name **ratio scale** reinforces the notion that *measurements obtained at this level and only at this level can be used to form ratios.* An ROM of 90 degrees is twice that of 45 degrees. A leg-length difference of 3 cm is half that of 6 cm. Measurements on the ratio scale can be subjected to addition, subtraction, multiplication, and division. If we measure the time it takes 25 patients with hemiplegia to walk a given distance, we can add the 25 measurements and divide the total by the number of patients (n=25) to compute the average or mean time for the group.

Interval Scales

Measurements on the interval scale are often used in physical therapy. An example is temperature (body, skin, whirlpool, hot pack, cold pack temperature, and so on) in degrees Fahrenheit or Celsius. Some developmental tests and many of the more recently developed tests of functional status are also considered interval scaled. Many psychological tests and measurements that are of interest to, but not administered by, physical therapists are examples of interval scales. Intelligence tests are usually considered interval in nature.

The interval scale is one in which the zero point does not represent an absence of the quantity being measured. This is sometimes mistakenly referred to as an "arbitrary" zero (as opposed to the "natural" zero of the ratio scale). Often the zero is far from arbitrary, as in the zero point on the Celsius scale, which reflects the temperature at which water freezes. The units on the interval scale must be of equal size. Because of the lack of a zero point, representing an absence of the quantity being measured, ratios should not be formed from measurements obtained using an interval scale.

Sometimes, the manner in which we obtain measurements creates the level of measurement. For example, torque is usually thought of as occurring on a ratio-scaled basis. There can be an absence of torque that represents a true zero. If a woman, however, extends her knee against the resistance of an isokinetic dynamometer, the only torque that is measured will be the torque the machine requires to keep the woman's limb from accelerating past the machine's speed setting. The torque the quadriceps femoris muscle needed to generate to move the limb up to that speed is not measured. The zero, therefore, does not represent an absence of torque generated by the quadriceps femoris muscle. Torques that have not been corrected for the effects of gravity (the missing torque in this example or the extra torque that occurs when movement is in the direction of gravity) should not be used to form ratios. The errors that occur in forming such ratios may be rather dramatic.

The following data, which are real and not hypothetical, show some of the potential pitfalls in creating ratios from uncorrected torques (interval-scaled data). Young women 25 to 34 years of age had their trunk flexor and extensor torques measured with an isokinetic device. The mean extensor torque was 82 Nm, and the mean flexor torque was 69 Nm. This would yield an extensor-to-flexor ratio of 1.18. When the torques are corrected for gravity, the mean values are 132 Nm and 48 Nm, respectively. This would yield a ratio of 2.75. There is more than a 100% error in this case when ratios are inappropriately formed from torques that were not gravity corrected. If the subjects, however, were able to generate less torque, the errors would be even greater. Older women (greater than 55 years of age) generated a mean of 56 Nm of extensor torque and a mean of 53 Nm of flexor torque, which yielded a non-gravity-corrected ratio of 1.05. Correction for the effect of gravity shows that extensor torque was 99 Nm and flexor torque was 30 Nm. The gravity-corrected "true ratio-scaled data" would yield an extensor-to-flexor ratio of 3.30. Here, the error is in excess of 300% (Sandler RB, Young RM, Delitto A, Burdett R; unpublished research). When interval-scaled data are used to form ratios, the errors are not always this dramatic, but some error will always occur, and test users need to judge whether this error is consequential.

The above example illustrates how important it is to know the level of measurement used and not to violate the rules associated with the use of that level of measurement. Measurements with errors of the types illustrated above can certainly lead to incorrect clinical decision making.

Most experts believe that interval-scaled measurements can be subjected to addition and subtraction. But the greatest proportion of experts use interval-scaled measurements in almost all types of mathematical calculations except for the formation of ratios. Sometimes, we forget that a percentage is a form of a ratio. Interval-scaled measurements should not, therefore, be used to generate percentages. For example, with the use of isokinetic dynamometers, it would be incorrect to describe one limb as generating a percentage of the torque generated by another limb unless both torque values were first gravity corrected to form ratio-scaled measurements.

An attribute represented on an interval scale can have, but need not have, a negative or minus value, as in the expression "-10° F." An attribute represented on a ratio scale cannot have negative or minus values.

Ordinal Scales

Examples of measurements on the ordinal scale in physical therapy are MMT grades, scores on some ADL tests, grades for various tests of neuro-motor performance (eg, Fugl-Meyer), and grades for most manual therapy and orthopedic tests (eg, tests of joint laxity and manual tests of ligamentous integrity).

Attributes measured by the use of ordinal scales are assigned a number or to a category that represents order or rank. The relative magnitude of the attribute is reflected in the ordering of the numerals, letters, or words assigned to describe the attribute. In its simplest form, an ordinal scale may have only two categories, representing the presence and the absence of something. There may or may not be an underlying assumption that one of the categories is *better* than the other, but there must be a contention that one or more of the categories reflect a greater quantity of what is being assessed. For example, **Independent** and **Dependent** in performing some activity are categories in which one appears better than the other. The two categories in this instance represent an order in that Independent is certainly "better than" Dependent. The presence and absence of an attribute can also be ordered so that the absence is better than the presence, as when the attribute is a disease, an injury, or a disability.

Ordinal scales usually have more than two categories. The number of categories on an ordinal scale is limited by the conceptual and practical difficulties in operationally defining different categories that could be logically ordered. The MMT grade of Good must be operationally defined as being distinctly different from and better than the grade of **Fair**. Some argue that this may not be possible because of the vagueness of the operational definitions for grades greater than Fair. Consider, however, the added difficulty of differentiating among grades when the same difference in muscle performance can be graded along an ordinal scale with pluses and minuses. In this case, instead of one differentiation being made (ie, between Good and Fair), a rater must differentiate among six categories: Fair minus, Fair, Fair plus, Good minus, Good, and Good plus. An ordinal scale, for example, with 20 categories requires some clever thinking to generate 20 distinctly different, ordered operational definitions that could be consistently followed.

The definitional requirements of ordinal scales are always more demanding than those of ratio or interval scales. Defining 1 cm on a ratio scale eliminates the need to define 2 cm, 3 cm, 4 cm, and so forth. Consider, for example, the challenge of classifying the severity of a low back injury, the level of disability due to a CVA, or the rehabilitation potential of a child with cystic fibrosis.

Some ordinal scales have numerals assigned as labels to their mutually exclusive and exhaustive categories. For example, MMT grades may be labeled 5 for Normal, 4 for Good, 3 for Fair, 2 for Poor, 1 for Trace, and 0 for Zero. The numerals 5, 4, 3, 2, 1, and 0 indicate order only, just as the words Normal, Good, Fair, Poor, Trace, and Zero indicate order only. The numerals do not indicate quantity; they have no numerical meaning other than order, and they should not be subjected to any mathematical operations. Ordinal data from a group can be characterized by use of the **mode** (most frequently occurring score) and the **median** (the middle value in the distribution).

The ordinal character of the numerals and words assigned to MMT grades is also not changed into a quantitative scale when the six categories are labeled as 100% (Normal), 80% (Good), 50% (Fair), 20% (Poor), 5% (Trace), and 0% (Zero). The percentage labels in this case indicate order only; they have no mathematical basis, and they can be misleading. The flaw in the percentage scheme is in thinking or advocating, for example, that a grade of Fair somehow represents 50% of what the grade of Normal represents (given that Normal is 100% of something). The point is belabored here to emphasize the limitations of ordinal scales. Ultimately, the real concern should be with the interpretations of measurements and the uses to which they are put. This concern begins to enter the arena of **validity**, a topic we will take up later in the *Primer*.

When an ordinal scale is used to test for an attribute in two or more persons, the summary data consist of the *counts of people* who have an attribute described by a category on the scale. These counts are called **frequency data**. Frequency data in the various categories on an ordinal scale can be added, and the sums in the categories can be expressed as percentages or proportions of the total number of all persons tested. You can say 20% of your patients, for example, have quadriceps femoris muscle MMT grades of Fair.

Nominal Scales

Examples of measurements on the nominal scale in physical therapy are categorization by disease types (eg, type of arthritis), type of low back disorder, type of amputation, type of cerebral palsy (CP), and type of breath sound.

In nominal scales, the units are categories that represent differences on an attribute without indicating the order or rank of the differences. These categories may be labeled with numerals, letters, or words, but regardless of how they are labeled, the labels do not indicate order or rank. In its simplest form, a nominal scale may have only two categories, representing the presence or the absence of an attribute.

Classifying by type of CP uses a nominal scale and is based on the premise that each type of CP is different than another. If the underlying assumption was that one category (ie, one type of CP) has more of some element than another, the scale would become, by definition, an ordinal scale. Nominal scales are used to differentiate people or things into groups based on definitions. Sometimes, we may have personal preferences about the groups, but that occurs outside of the scaling process. We may, for example, believe one type of CP is more amenable to treatment than another, but the classification is still nominal. Similarly, if we were to classify ice cream flavors, we may have a favorite among the classifications, but the process of classification is not based on implementing a value system, but rather solely on differentiation based on defined criteria (ie, the flavor).

The nominal scale is often said to represent the simplest form of measurement by permitting recognition of similarities and differences among people (or objects), classifying people (or objects) in categories according to their similarities and differences, and counting the number of instances in each category. Measurement, however, even in its simplest form, requires adherence to operational definitions and to mutually exclusive and exhaustive units or categories in the same manner as does measurement in any form.

Are There Good and Bad Levels of Measurements?

Often, experts on measurement will express a distinct bias that the best measurements are those made using ratio or interval scales. They would be aghast if any person used ratio- or interval-scaled data to make classifications, because they would argue that in the process of going from one scale to the other, information is lost. Their premise, however, may be fallacious. In clinical practice, ratio- and interval-scaled measurements are often taken for the purpose of making a decision, but that decision often represents using the data to assign the patient or an attribute to a nominal or ordinal category.

Even when measuring ROM in a patient with adhesive capsulitis, we will often be forced at various points during a treatment program to determine whether this patient is making significant enough progress to warrant continued treatment. We are, in effect, using the change in ROM, a ratio-scaled measurement, and classifying that change as being either acceptable or unacceptable, an ordinal-scaled measurement.

Clinical documentation and research that are reported only with the use of ratio- and interval-scaled measurements may provide information that does not really reflect clinically relevant issues. Reporting that an exercise program increases a muscle's torque production, for example, seems like a good thing. But if an average increase in torque for a group of patients was large because only the weakest subjects in a treatment group improved, we may erroneously deem a treatment as beneficial, because we looked at ratio-scaled data even though not one person receiving the treatment may have been classified as attaining a level of clinical success (categorical data). In this case, although the average may have increased, it is possible that no patients attained a high enough torque to become functional in an area in which they had previously lost function.

One of the benefits of interval- and ratio-scaled data, however, is that these data can often be used to reflect small changes in measurements, changes that might not affect group assignment or ranks. Ratio- and interval-scaled measurements may, therefore, be more sensitive in reflecting changes in a variable.

Levels of measurement are not inherently good or bad, desirable or undesirable. Ratio and interval scales may seem to provide more data. But, the real issue is: What information should the data convey? *The level of measurement should be chosen based on what needs to be measured and how the measurement will be used.* Ratio-scaled pulmonary function tests may indicate the type and intensity of intervention that is needed. On the other hand, classification of a person as being independent or dependent following a CVA (use of categorical data) carries a lot more information than do the person's torque and ROM values (ratio-scaled data).

Transformation of Scales

Ratio- and interval-scaled measurements can be aggregated into two or more categories so that, in effect, the scale is transformed into an ordinal scale. If, for example, we have measurements of right knee extensor isokinetic peak torque on 88 patients, we could compute the mean peak torque and then determine whose measurements were above the mean and whose were at or below the mean. By assigning each measurement to one of the two groups, we have created ordinal data from the ratio-scaled data. We also could have computed the median (the 50th percentile) and used it as the point at which to split the 88 patients into two ordinal-scaled groups of 50% each.

Measurements based on ratio or interval scales can be aggregated or "collapsed" into two or more categories on ordinal scales (as in the above example), in effect transforming the ratio or interval scale into an ordinal scale. This transformation does not actually transform the measurements. The effect on the measurements is one of *replacing* the original measurements, that is, the numerals that represented varying quantities on a ratio (or interval) scale, and *substituting* new measurements in the form of numerals that represent counts of people in categories on an ordinal scale. Transformation of a scale from a higher form (ratio or interval) to a lower form (ordinal) is legitimate, but it can have the effect of discarding valuable information on the variability of individual measurements. The transformation may also have a beneficial effect if it focuses the measurement in more relevant terms, for example, when deciding whether a person is ready to be progressed to the next level of exercise. A "yes" or "no" decision must be made; such a decision is really an ordinal classification. In this case, we might be using interval- or ratio-scaled torque measurements to make a "yes" or "no" (categorical) classification.

When a measurement is examined to determine whether it has the appropriate qualities (eg, reliability and validity), the final measurement should be examined, not those measurements that are used to derive or to lead to the final measurement. For example, if we wanted to determine whether an ordinal classification of patients with hemiplegia met the criteria outlined in the *Standards*, we would examine the classifications, not the interval- or ratio-scaled data that may have been used for classification (eg, time to put on clothes, distance walked).

Transformation of measurements can only be done in a way that reduces information. Transformation of ordinal- or nominal-scaled data into ratio- or interval-scaled data is never appropriate.

Quantitative and Qualitative Scales

The four levels used for measurements are of two major kinds, namely, quantitative and qualitative.

Quantitative scales are scales on which the defined units are assumed to be of equal size and to represent quantities of the attribute or underlying phenomenon. There appears to be universal agreement that the **ratio** scale is a quantitative scale. A measurement based on a quantitative scale is expressed as a quantity **of something**. A "10" on a quantitative scale is **10 of something**: 10 cm of length, 10 milliseconds of time, or 10 mg of weight. **Interval** scales are also quantitative scales.

If the quantitative scale is also a **continuous** scale, the equal-sized units on the scale can be subdivided into equal-sized subunits. Those subunits can then be subdivided still further into equal-sized subunits. For example, the meter can be subdivided into centimeters, which can be subdivided even further into millimeters, and so on.

If the quantitative scale is not continuous, then it is discrete. The units on a scale that is quantitative and discrete represent nondivisible entities. A count of people is a ratio-scaled measurement, expressed as a whole number, that represents a quantity of discrete, indivisible entities. One cannot count 6.75 people. One may see an average of 6.75 patients per day, but one cannot see 6.75 patients on a given day.

Qualitative scales are scales in which the defined categories have no known size or are assumed to have no size, and therefore cannot represent quantities. Attributes measured with qualitative scales cannot be assumed to be of equal size and are not divisible into equal-sized subcategories. Qualitative scales are used to test qualities, not quantities, of an attribute. The categories on a qualitative scale that is also ordinal indicate relative order on the attribute to which the scale applies. Deep tendon reflexes, for example, can be assessed with the categories Zero (areflexia), Plus (hyporeflexia), 1 to 3 (average), and 3+ and 4+ (hyperreflexive). These grades are supposed to indicate qualitative, nonquantitative differences in reflex activity. Zero is different from Plus, and 1 is different from 3+. The grades reflect the relative order of the gradations of reflex activity. Sitting balance, levels of ambulatory independence, and MMT grades are other examples of qualitative categorizations based on ordinal ranks.

The categories on a qualitative scale that is also **nominal** (not ordinal) are assumed to indicate only nonquantitative differences, not relative order, on the attribute to which the scale applies. In classifying patients according to diagnosis, the categories indicate nonquantitative differences only (the presence of different qualities), not relative order.

Fundamental and Derived Measurements

Fundamental measurements are those that are obtained initially without the need for derivation. Leg length represents a fundamental measurement that is used to derive the measurement of leg-length difference. The measurement of leg-length differences, for example, is derived by subtracting one leg-length measurement from another. A derived measurement is defined in the Standards as "a measurement of an attribute that is obtained as the result of a mathematical operation applied to an existing measurement."*

Another derived measurement is the motor nerve conduction velocity. In this case, we derive a measurement from a derived measurement. First, the examiner determines the latency (time) between stimulation and arrival of a potential at two points along the course of a nerve. Measurements of latency are fundamental, not derived. The conduction time, which is determined by subtracting one latency from the other, is a **derived measurement**. This derived measurement is then used to determine conduction velocity (in meters per second) by dividing the distance (in millimeters) between the two points of stimulation by the conduction time (in milliseconds).

Derived measurements, logically conceived, have an important place in identifying, defining, and testing attributes that are conceptually and theoretically essential to an area of practice or science. Derived measurements can represent the practical effects of insight and abstraction. Very often, derived measurements represent the use of measurements of one attribute to create measurements of a different attribute. Measurements of time and linear distances were used, for example, to create a measurement of conduction velocity. The creation of derived measurements is beneficial when it helps represent phenomena that are of interest.

Change Measurements (Scores)

Measurements can be used to represent changes in people when they are tested on two or more occasions over time. A **change measurement** consists of the mathematical difference between two of the same kinds of measurements taken on the same person at two different points in time. The action of choosing to use a change measurement (instead of, for example, the obtained measurement at time 1 and the obtained measurement at time 2) is really one of *redefining* the attribute to be measured. Change measurements, as *measurements in their own right*, are fraught with theoretical and conceptual problems that exceed the complexities addressed in this *Primer*.[9-12] This does not mean, however, that change measurements do not have potential value, particularly in clinical practice. Users of change scores should be aware of the problems associated with this type of score and exercise caution in making conclusions based on change scores.

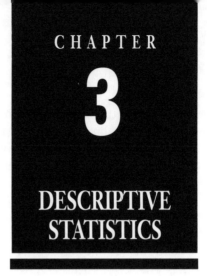

S tatistics are discussed in this *Primer* because basic concepts related to statistics are essential to understanding and using measurements. This is especially true when discussing reliability and validity of measurements, and when using normative values.

A **statistic** is a single numerical value or index, derived from a set of measurements. Statistics may summarize or describe all members of a group on an attribute, dimension, or variable. A **descriptive statistic** is a statistic that is a single numerical value or index, derived from a set of measurements, that summarizes or describes members of a group on an attribute. **Inferential statistics** are based on measurements obtained from samples and are used to reflect characteristics of a population. Inferential statistics may be used on data from a sample to estimate descriptive statistics for a population, to determine whether sets of data are different or the same, or to determine whether sets of data are mathematically related.

Mean, Median, Mode, and Distributions

(Measures of Central Tendency)

The **mean** or **arithmetic average** of a series of quantitative measurements is a statistic. Contrary to popular biases, statistics make life easier, not more complex. Statistics can be useful, for example, when we try to understand measurements of passive right hip flexion in male patients, aged 59 to 75 years, with osteoarthritis. If there were only 3 patients, we could summarize or describe all the members of the group by simply citing the hip flexion measurements for each of the 3 patients. We might do the same thing if there were 10 patients, but the task could become more difficult. Trying to keep in mind measurements from 10 people simultaneously could be overwhelming.

If there were 30 patients, or 100 patients, or 300 patients, citing the hip flexion measurements for each patient would be almost impossible. Statistics allow us to summarize or describe all the members of a group when it is not possible (practical) to deal with individual measurements. The mean of the 30, 100, or 300 measurements serves to describe the *average amount* of maximal right hip flexion in these patients, and could be used to provide a comparison between hip flexion in this group and hip flexion in a comparable group of male patients, aged 59 to 75 years, who do not have osteoarthritis. Such comparisons are virtually impossible without appropriate statistics such as the mean.

The mean is one **measure of central tendency** (measure of central location). The **median**, the middle value in a distribution of measurements (scores), is another measure of central tendency. The median is the statistic that describes the **midpoint among a number of quantitative measurements** in a set of measurements. If, for example, passive-range-of-motion (PROM) measurements of right hip flexion were available on 30 patients, the median would be the point (expressed in degrees of flexion) above which no more than 15 of the patients would have measurements and below which no more than 15 of the patients would have measurements.

Because the median is the measurement that attempts to divide all measurements into an upper 50% and a lower 50%, another name for the median is the 50th percentile, the point below which 50% of the measurements occur.

The **mode** is also a statistical measure of **central tendency** or **central location.** The mode is the value obtained most often. The value of the mode is *not* computed arithmetically, but it is obtained by observing the frequency distribution of a set of measurements.

The three measures of *central tendency each provide different insights.* The *mean* has to do with the actual quantities of the attribute measured. The *median* splits a set of measurements into two equal-sized groups. The *mode* reflects what is the most frequently obtained measurement.

If the frequencies of all obtained measurements are plotted on a graph, they would form a curve (frequency along the Y-axis [the ordinate] and measurement values along the X-axis [the abscissa]). A normal curve is a hypothetical, symmetrical, bell-shaped graphic representation of how the distribution of measurements would look if an infinite number of measurements could be obtained. Many of the attributes measured by physical therapists will be distributed along a normal curve if enough measurements are obtained. Most of the measurements would be clustered in or near the middle. The measurements with high numerical values and low numerical values would be spread rather evenly on both sides of the middle, and only a few measurements will have very high or very low values.

Measurement of Hip Abduction Range of Motion (°)	Healthy Adults	Young Athletes	Elderly Patients	Patients Following a Total Hip Replacement
65	2	10	2	6
60	4	12	2	10
55	6	8	2	6
50	8	6	2	2
45	10	6	6	2
40	8	2	6	2
35	6	2	8	6
30	4	2	12	10
25	2	2	10	6
Total Number of Persons in Each Group	50	50	50	50

Table 1. Four Distributions of Measurements on Groups of 50 Hypothetical Patients

If the mean, median, and mode are close together in the distribution of measurement values, it is reasonable to conclude that the distribution of the measurements in the population is essentially **normal,** and that if the distribution of measurements were graphed, a bell-shaped curve would be formed.

Some measurements do **not** peak in the center of the distribution of measurements. Measurements may peak at one end or the other of the distribution; that is, there are more high values or more low values. Measurements may even peak at *two* or more places in the distribution. A distribution that has two distinct modes is called **bimodal.**

Some distributions of measurements are illustrated in figures based on data from Table 1. The table contains hypothetical data on hip abduction ROM values taken from four different groups with each representing a different distribution.

In the first example, the healthy adults (illustrated in Fig. 1), there are more measurements of patients at and near the middle of the measurement values (10 patients received a measurement value of 45, 8 patients

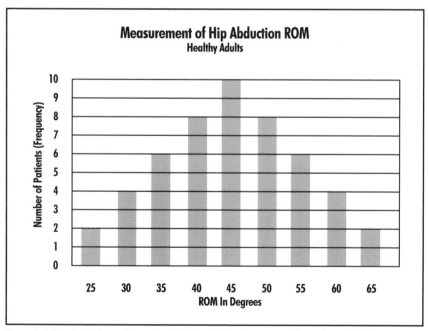

Figure 1. This depiction of hypothetical hip abduction range-of-motion (ROM) measurements in healthy adults approximates a normal distribution.

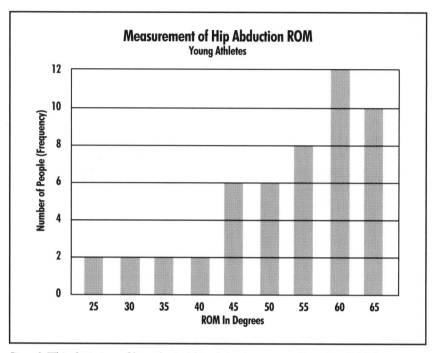

Figure 2. This depiction of hypothetical hip abduction range-of-motion (ROM) measurements approximates a negatively (left) skewed distribution with a left tail.

received a value of 50, and 8 patients received a value of 40). There are also fewer measurements at the two ends of the distribution (2 patients received a value of 65, 4 patients received a value of 60, 4 patients received a value of 30, and 2 patients received a value of 25). The frequency of measurements *peaked at the center and tapered off symmetrically toward each end.*

The distribution does not form a perfectly normal distribution, but it comes very close. One would guess, for example, that if more and more patients' ROM was measured, the resulting distribution would even more closely approach a normal distribution.

The mode for the healthy adults is 45 because the measurement value of 45 is the value obtained most frequently (by 10 patients). We will see later that in a distribution that closely resembles a normal distribution, the mean, the median, and the mode will be essentially in the same place and will have essentially the same value.

In the second example, the young athletes (illustrated in Fig. 2), most of the 50 patients' measurements have high values at and near the values of 65 and 60. The distribution shown for the young athletes is called a **skewed** distribution, meaning that the distribution is lopsided or asymmetrical and does not resemble the normal curve. The peaking is at one end, not in or near the center, and there is an absence of symmetrical tapering off in both directions from the peak. Indeed, the only tapering off is toward the low end of the measurement values. The *skewing of the distribution is named according to the direction of the long tail.* In this example, the distribution is negatively skewed.

The mode for the young athletes is 60 (that is, the value of 60 was obtained most frequently). The median (55) is pulled away just slightly from the mode and toward the long tail of this skewed distribution. The mean (52.8) is pulled away even farther than the median from the mode and toward the long tail of the distribution. In other words, *the mean of a skewed distribution of measurement values will be affected more than the median by the few extreme measurement values in the long tail of the distribution.* The mean is more labile than the median in the face of extreme measurements.

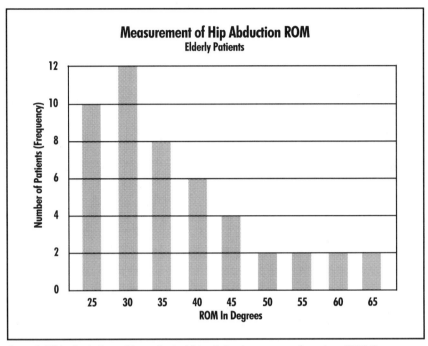

Figure 3. This depiction of hypothetical hip abduction range-of-motion (ROM) measurements approximates a positively (right) skewed distribution with a right tail.

In the third example, the elderly patients (illustrated in Fig. 3), the measurements reflect a reversal of the distribution seen for the young athletes. Most of the 50 measurements are at the low end. Everything said about the distribution for the young athletes can be said about the distribution for the elderly group, except that the distribution is *positively* skewed with a right tail.

The mode is 30. The median (35) is pulled away just slightly from the mode and toward the long tail of this skewed distribution. The mean (37.2) is pulled away farther than the median from the mode and toward the long tail of this distribution. In other words, the mean of a skewed distribution of measurement values will be affected more than the median by the few extreme measurement values in the tail of the distribution. The mean is more affected than the median by extreme measurements.

The fourth example, the measurements taken postoperatively from patients receiving total hip replacements (illustrated in Fig. 4), presents a different situation. The distribution has *two* modes (one at 30 and one at 60) and no tapering off in either direction. The distribution has symmetry, but not the pattern of symmetry that typifies the curve describing the normal distribution. Because it has two modes, the distribution illustrated in Figure 4 is called bimodal.

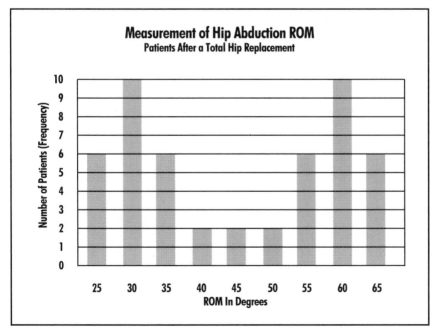

Figure 4. The depiction of hypothetical hip abduction range-of-motion (ROM) measurements illustrates a bimodal distribution.

One possible interpretation of a bimodal distribution is that the group or sample measured may have actually consisted of persons from two different populations. Often, no attempt is made to compute, report, and interpret the mean and median on a distribution of measurements that is bimodal because these indices of central tendency, quite literally, would have no centrality to which they could logically refer. A statistic designed to summarize or describe the central tendency of measurements for all of the members of a group will make no sense if the group has no central tendency.

Among the three measures of central tendency (mean, median, mode), the mean is often the preferred statistic because (1) it represents the average quantity and (2) it has mathematical properties that enable the use of statistical methods. *The mean is the midway point among the numerical values of the measurements.* The mean of a set of quantitative measurements is operationally defined as the sum or total of the numerical values of the measurements divided by the number of measurements.

COMPUTING THE MEAN

Mean = Sum of Measurements/Number of Measurements

Table 2. Hypothetical Data to Illustrate the Properties of the Mean

Measurements	Measurement - Mean (DEVIATION SCORE)
7	7 - 5 = 2
7	7 - 5 = 2
7	7 - 5 = 2
6	6 - 5 = 1
6	6 - 5 = 1
6	6 - 5 = 1
THE MEAN (5) IS THE MIDPOINT	SUM OF DEVIATIONS ABOVE THE MEAN = +9
4	4 - 5 = -1
3	3 - 5 = -2
3	3 - 5 = -2
1	1 - 5 = -4
Sum = 50	0
N = 10	SUM OF DEVIATIONS BELOW THE MEAN = -9
Mean = 50/10 = 5	

In the example shown in Table 2, the mean or arithmetic average is 5.00. For convenience, the 10 measurement values have been listed in order from highest to lowest.

The sum of deviations (the differences between the mean and the measurements) above the mean is +9. The sum of deviation scores below the mean is -9. When the deviations from the mean are computed as shown in Table 2, the sum of the deviations above the mean will equal the sum of the deviations below the mean, and the total of all of the deviations will be zero. By definition, this characteristic of the mean is always true.

If the attribute measured has some scores that are much higher or much lower than most of the scores, the mean will tend to be pulled away from the greater number of measurements. The mean will move away from the median. We can use the same hypothetical measurements of hip abduction ROM that we previously discussed to further describe properties of the mean, the median, and the mode.

Measurements of Hip Abduction ROM (°)	Healthy Adults (Frequency for Each Measurement)	Frequency x Measurement	Young Athletes (Frequency for Each Measurement)	Frequency x Measurement	Elderly Patients (Frequency for Each Measurement)	Frequency x Measurement
25	2	50	2	50	10	250
30	4	120	2	60	12	360
35	6	210	2	70	8	280
40	8	320	2	80	6	240
45	10	450	6	270	6	270
50	8	400	6	300	2	100
55	6	330	8	440	2	110
60	4	240	12	720	2	120
65	2	130	10	650	2	130
Sum	50	2,250	50	2,640	50	1,860
Mean		45		52.8		37.2
Median		45		55		35
Mode		45		60		30

Table 3. Hypothetical Range-of-Motion (ROM) Data Illustrating Properties of the Mean, Median, and Mode

Table 3 contains measurements that are essentially normally distributed (healthy adults), negatively skewed (young athletes), and positively skewed (elderly patients). To simplify the table, we did not use each subject's measurements. Instead, we showed the frequency of occurrence of each measurement. We multiplied each measurement by the number of subjects who had that measurement (the score x the frequency of occurrence) in order to calculate a mean.

In examining the table, there may be a tendency to focus on the three means (45, 52.8, and 37.2). Given that most measurements are in the mid-range of values for the healthy adults, at the high end for the young athletes, and at the low end for the elderly patients, the three means each are affected differently by the three different distributions. The mean for the normally distributed values for the healthy adults lies in the center of the distribution. The mean for the young athletes with their frequently occurring high score is moved to the right or upward. The mean for the elderly patients with their frequently occurring low scores is moved to the left or downward. This illustrates that, with a skewed distribution the mean moves and becomes a less useful measure of central tendency than when measurements are normally distributed.

For the normally distributed measurements taken from the healthy adults, all three measures of central tendency, the mean, the median, and the mode, are the same. This is in contrast to what can be seen for the young athletes, whose values for the three measurements of central tendency are not the same. The distribution is negatively skewed, with most of the measurements at the higher values, and with a long, tapering tail toward the lower values. The skewing pulls the median slightly away from the mode and toward the tail, and pulls the mean farther away from the mode and toward the tail. The mode is 60 and "follows the crowd," so to speak. The median is 55, and the mean of 52.8 is being dragged downward by the long tail. The mean, despite being the preferred measure of central tendency, varies greatly as a function of extreme scores. The data from the elderly adults demonstrate the effects of a skewed distribution on measures of central tendency, but show the opposite effects seen in the data from the young athletes.

The median is often the preferred measure of central tendency when there is concern that measurements are severely skewed. There are methods for quantifying the degree of skewedness of a distribution (just as there are methods for quantifying the flatness or "peakedness" of a distribution [measurements of **kurtosis**]),[13,14] but this information often is not used in deciding whether to use the mean instead of the median to describe central tendencies. The decision depends on the use to which the mean or median will be put, the interpretation to be put on that use of the mean or median, the nature of the attribute being measured, the sample that was measured, and the number of measurements. A sensible rule of thumb is this: When in doubt, examine both the mean and the median.

The mean is often more easily and meaningfully interpreted when it is accompanied by the **standard deviation** and the **variance**, two measurements of variability that will be described in other sections of the *Primer*. The best way to describe data is often to report the mean, the standard deviation, and the range of values.

Distributions may also be effectively characterized by reporting measurements in terms of percentiles. The median is, by definition, the measurement that falls into the 50th percentile; it is the measurement below which no more than 50% of the measurements occur. The 90th percentile is that measurement point below which 90% of the measurements occur, the 75th percentile is that measurement point below which 75% of the measurements occur, and so forth.

Percentiles allow for rapid evaluation of how a measurement compares with other measurements taken from a sample. Knowing that a healthy adult has 60 degrees of hip abduction ROM provides some information, but it would also be useful to know that the measurement places the person in the 90th percentile. In other words, 90% of those measured would have less ROM. Unfortunately, we do not now have data to make that type of comparison. **Normative data** are more easily interpreted when the data are accompanied by measures of **central tendency**, **measures of variability**, and descriptions of **percentiles**.

Variance and Standard Deviation

(Measures of Variability)

When quantitative measurements are available, the measures of central tendency, the mean and the median, are useful but not sufficient for describing the group as a whole. Summarizing or describing the measurements for a group by use of the mean says nothing about **variability**, or how measurements differ from each other. Because the sum of deviations from the mean is, by definition, zero, other methods must be used to describe variability. There are two commonly used statistics that describe how much variability there is in a set of measurements: the **variance** and the **standard deviation**. The two statistics are related because the standard deviation is the square root of the variance.

Measurements	Deviations (MEASUREMENT - THE MEAN)	Deviations Squared
7	$7 - 5 = 2$	4
7	$7 - 5 = 2$	4
7	$7 - 5 = 2$	4
6	$6 - 5 = 1$	1
6	$6 - 5 = 1$	1
6	$6 - 5 = 1$	1
4	$4 - 5 = -1$	1
3	$3 - 5 = -2$	4
3	$3 - 5 = -2$	4
1	$1 - 5 = -4$	16
Sum = 50	Sum = 0	40 Sum of the Squared Deviations
N = 10		
Mean = 5		
Population Variance = 40/10 = 4		
Population Standard Deviation $=\sqrt{4} = 2$		

Table 4. Deviations From the Mean as a Source of Variance

The **variance** is the average squared deviation (difference) from the mean. *Table 4 illustrates how the variance and the standard deviation are calculated when all subjects in a population have been measured.* Rarely, however, do we have the chance to measure all subjects in a population. When measurements are obtained from a sample, a different calculation is used.

The **population variance** is the **mean squared deviation**. In our example, the population variance is 4.00 and the population standard deviation is the square root of the variance (the square root of 4.00 is 2.00). *Without variance, the mean of a set of measurements has no context within which it can be judged.* A mean alone does not really characterize a set of measurements unless it is accompanied by the variance or the standard deviation. Table 4 demonstrates two ideas: (1) that the deviation for each measurement is obtained by subtracting the mean from each measurement and (2) that the sum of the deviations is zero.

Formulas for Calculating the Population Variance and Population Standard Deviation

Population Variance for a Set of Measurements =   Sum of Squared Deviations Divided by Number of Measurements

Population Variance for Measurements in Table 4 = $40 \div 10 = 4$

Population Standard Deviation for Measurements in Table 4 = Square Root of Variance

Population Standard Deviation for Measurements in Table 4 = $\sqrt{4} = 2$

The size of the variance can vary. Figure 5 illustrates hypothetical measurements taken on 50 people, and in each case the distribution approximates a normal curve (ie, most of the measurements are in the middle of each distribution). Each distribution is also symmetrical (the numbers of measurements taper off more or less sharply in both directions from the middle of each distribution), and the mean, median, and mode are in the same place in each distribution. The mean in each case is 5.00.

Distribution 1 has approximately the amount of peaking in the middle and tapering toward the ends that would be expected with a normal distribution. The peaking in distribution 2 is even more pronounced, and there is little tapering toward the ends. Distribution 3 appears almost flat, with a small hump in the middle and with tapering off toward the ends (eg, fewer scores toward the ends).

Distributions may vary in "peakedness" or flatness. **Kurtosis** (from the Greek *kyrtósis* for convexity or **curvature**) is a measure that reflects the peakedness of a curve (eg, the greater the peak, the greater the kurtosis). The *sharply peaked* distribution (distribution 2) is called a **leptokurtic distribution**. The *relatively flat* distribution shown for distribution 3 is called a **platykurtic distribution**. An *absolutely flat* distribution is a **rectangular distribution**.

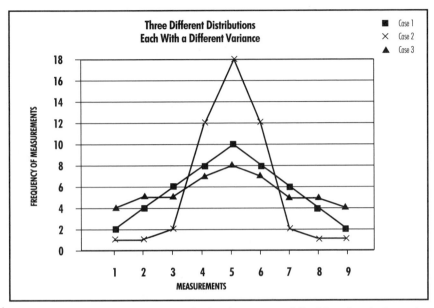

Figure 5. Each distribution has a mean of 5, but the variances differ. Note that the lower the peak of the curve, the greater the variance. The more scores that are bunched toward the mean, the lower the variance.

Most professional and scientific journals and measurement handbooks will not publish tables of raw data (ie, every measurement obtained). Tables of raw data (individual measurements) consume too much space to warrant their publication. Therefore, use of measures of central tendency combined with measures of variability are the only way in which a reader can discern the true nature of a distribution when that distribution is not presented graphically or in the form of raw data. The prevailing custom is to report the standard deviation along with the mean for a set of measurements. The range would also be useful and is required in the journal *Physical Therapy*.

The standard deviation is often used to make decisions about measurements. When measurements from a population are normally distributed, approximately 34% of all measurements will be within 1 standard deviation of the mean. Or when expressed in terms of variability, approximately 68% of the measurements will be within ± 1 standard deviation from the mean (34% for 1 standard deviation above and 34% for 1 standard deviation below) (Fig. 6).

The normal distribution is marked by a moderate amount of piling up of measurements in and near the middle of the distribution, with the number of measurements tapering off toward the higher and lower measurement values at each end of the distribution. Although the first standard deviation above the mean includes approximately 34% of the measurements in a normal distribution, the second standard deviation above the mean includes approximately just an additional 14% of the measurements. Therefore, ± 2 standard deviations will encompass approximately, for scores above the mean, 14%+34%=48% and, for measurements below the mean, 14%+34%=48%, a total of 96% of all measurements.

The implication is clear. If a score is *more* than 2 standard deviations *above* the mean or *more* than 2 standard deviations *below* the mean, that score has only a 4% chance of coming from the population from which the distribution was derived. Someone who obtains that score may or may not belong to the population, but no matter what, the person is clearly in the minority within that population relative to the variable being measured. The standard deviation is important in the interpretation of normative data and will be further discussed along with that topic.

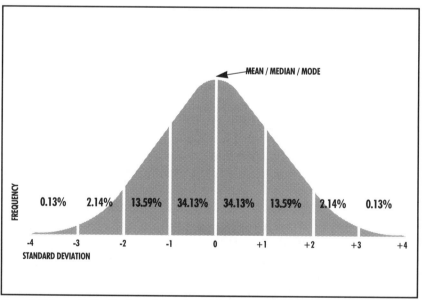

Figure 6. "Normal" distribution of data, in which the mean, the median, and the mode are all the same. Note the percentages of measurements that fall within each standard deviation from the mean.

Samples, Populations, Estimates, and Parameters

In measuring an attribute from a group of patients of a particular kind (who, because of their unique identity, may be considered a group), the measurements obtained are descriptive for that group. Often, someone will propose that a *group* of patients is somehow *representative* of patients of *a particular kind*. When this occurs, the measurements obtained from *that group* tend to be *generalized* to other patients of that particular kind. This includes *patients of that kind who have never been seen and who may never be seen*. Because we can never hope to see all patients of a given kind, we must learn from previous experience with patients to project what is learned into expectations, anticipations, plans, and actions concerning patients *not yet seen*. The behavior is not only proper, it is essential if one is to practice. The logic in generalizing measurements obtained on a group of patients **(a sample)** to a larger group **(a population)** is sound, and there are inferential statistics that can be used when these generalizations are needed.

If generalization to a population is going to occur, an operational definition of the patient population must exist before a sample of patients can be measured. Will the patient population be all patients with hemiplegia? Or patients with left hemiplegia only? Of any ages, or of specified ages? Of both genders? Only when we are satisfied with the operational definition of the patient population, and the **representativeness** of the patient group in the sample, should measurements be used to calculate the **sample mean (the average of all scores obtained in the sample).** The sample mean is called the **best estimate** of the population mean. The sample mean, unlike other sample statistics (the sample variance and sample standard deviation), is calculated using the same formula as is used for the population statistic.

If a colleague agrees to use your operational definition for the same patient population, and agrees to obtain the same measurement, in the same way, on the same size sample of patients representing the same population, will you both obtain the same sample mean? Probably not! The sample mean you obtained and the sample mean your colleague obtains, however, are *both* best estimates of the population mean. If you both measure small numbers of patients, your means may differ greatly. But, if you both measure large numbers of patients, your estimates of the population mean improve (both more closely approximate the true mean), and as a result the two sample means are likely to become closer.

You and your colleague may want to pool your measurements to obtain one best estimate of the population mean. The principle may be extended to include the cooperation of colleagues in a number of states and countries. Whatever the size of the sample, it would still be a sample of the patient population, and the resulting mean(s) would be sample mean(s). The larger the sample size, the closer the sample mean will get to the true population mean. The sample mean, therefore, is an approximation of the population mean and becomes a better approximation with increased sample size. All inferential statistics that examine data from samples better reflect the population when the sample size increases.

We can now extend the explanation to the **sample variance** and the sample **standard deviation**. If the variance or standard deviation for a sample are calculated using the forms of those statistics designed to describe populations, they provide a **biased estimate** of the population variance and population standard deviation. The formulas for calculating population variance and population standard deviation will lead to underestimates of the true values when they are used on samples.

To get the **best estimate** of the population variance from a sample, there is a very practical and simple way of correcting the sample variance.

Formulas for Calculating the Sample Variance and Sample Standard Deviation

Sample Variance for a Set of Measurements = Sum of Deviations Squared/(Number of Measurements-1)

Sample Variance for a Set of Measurements = $40 \div (10 - 1) = 4.44$

Sample Standard Deviation for a Set of Measurements = Square Root of Sample Variance

Sample Standard Deviation for a Set of Measurements = $\sqrt{4.44} = 2.107$

The correction is to divide the sum of deviations squared by the number of measurements minus one (n-1) instead of just the number of measurements. *The population variance in our example is 4.00*, and the *sample* variance is *4.44*. The correction takes the population variance and *increases* its size somewhat to provide an estimate of the population variance when only a sample is measured. The correction of the denominator for computing sample variance will have a greater effect on samples of small size than on samples of large size. Suppose, for example, that the sum of the squared deviations from the mean were 40 and N (the number of measurements) were 4:

Population Variance=40/4=10.00
Sample Variance=40/(4-1)=40/3=13.33

Now, if the sum of the squared deviations from the mean were 400 and there were 40 measurements (N=40):

Population Variance=400/40=10.00
Sample Variance=400/(40-1)=400/39=10.03

In the second example with the larger sample size, the population and sample variances were much closer. *Small samples, therefore, have more variance simply as a function of sample size, and the estimates of standard deviation and variance will be large to compensate for the sample size.* With small sample sizes, generalizations to populations are difficult and more error-ridden than with large sample sizes.

The word **parameter** is the generic name that is applied to the mean, the variance, or the standard deviation of a population. A parameter is a single, numerical value or index that summarizes all of the members of a population relative to an attribute. A parameter can only be estimated from a sample statistic; it cannot be obtained from a sample.

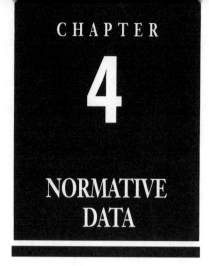

CHAPTER

4

NORMATIVE DATA

One way in which measurements may be interpreted is by comparing a given measurement with those obtained from other persons. How do we choose which scores to compare with? If we want to make judgments about whether a value is good or bad, acceptable or unacceptable, indicative or nonindicative of pathology, we might choose to compare with a measurement obtained from a specific person. For example, if we are attempting to rehabilitate a hurdler, we might want to compare the lower-extremity ROM measurements of our patient with those of a person capable of running the hurdles. Such a comparison uses what is called a **criterion reference** (ie, a score is compared with another score that is known to be good). The **criterion** is the measurement that is held up as the **standard.** There is essentially a judgment that some value is good or bad. Criterion referencing will be discussed in greater detail later.

A second way in which we make judgments about measurements is to determine how a given score compares with those we would expect to find in the population of interest. This is called **normative referencing**. The word **normative** refers not to a judgment of good or bad, or healthy or desirable, but rather to the use of the normal distribution.

Normative data (norms) can be used to see how an individual's measurement "stacks up" with respect to measurements of the same attribute obtained from a relevant population. In order to make such comparisons, we need **norms** in the form of normative data and **normative descriptive statistics** for measurements of the attribute from the relevant population.

The following scenario provides some insights into the use of normative data. Mrs Jones is a 73-year-old, white, female, retired accountant who complains of general joint stiffness and pain that is worse in the mornings, on cloudy and rainy days, and after long automobile trips to visit her grandchildren. When walking, her stance time for her right lower extremity is less than for her left. Her step length is shorter on the left than on the right. Her right knee is kept in a position of about 20 degrees of flexion during stance. In going up and down steps, she obviously "favors" her right knee by relying on the use of a handrail when bearing weight on the right lower extremity. Goniometric measurements of her knees show a PROM of 20 to 100 degrees of flexion on the right and 10 to 120 degrees of flexion on the left. *How do Mrs Jones' goniometric measurements compare with respect to what should be expected for her age, her gender, her occupation, and her likely diagnosis?*

If you answered the question, on what basis did you answer? How do you know what should be expected: From your own experience? By the motion available in your own knees? From the advice of your former instructor, from notes taken when you were a student? Perhaps you answered on the basis of the average ROM for the knee as published in the *International SFTR Method of Measuring and Recording Joint Motion*[15] or some other book. If the latter, how, where, and on whom did the authors of that text obtain their "averages"? Or, by chance, did you know what should be expected because you consulted your own copy of the *Worldwide Almanac of Norms and Normative Data and Statistics for Goniometric Measurements of Passive and Active Motion in Human Axial and Appendicular Skeleton Joints—Organized According to Age, Gender, Occupation, the Top Twenty Most Common Diagnoses Affecting Joint Motion, and Other Miscellaneous Factors?* If you answered "yes" to the last question, let us know where you got the publication and how much it cost! We know of no sources other than our imaginary almanac that actually provide normative data for ROM in a way that meets routine statistical requirements.

With very few exceptions, physical therapy does not yet have a supply of norms in the form of normative data and normative descriptive statistics on the attributes and the populations that are germane to the field. The *Standards* state that test developers, promoters, and sellers should provide manuals that include normative data. In addition, the *Standards* specify how such data should be described and the circumstances under which the data should be collected. Consider how much easier clinical decision making might be if normative data were available. Consider how much easier it might be to justify treatment to governmental agencies and third-party payers if such data were available for comparisons.

The following excerpt from the *Standards* describes and explains what is required if normative data are to be meaningful: *"P18.1. Descriptions of who obtained the normative data must be provided in the test manual."**

In order for normative data to have any meaning, a person using the data must know whether the measurements he or she obtains would be similar to those described by the normative data. If normative data were obtained by persons very skilled in obtaining measurements, only persons with similar skills could obtain measurements that should be compared. The real issue is comparability of data. The *Standards* state:

> **P18.4.** *Descriptions of persons who took the measurements used to obtain the normative data (ie, those who were in the role of test users) must be provided in the test manual. The test manual should include descriptions of test users' qualifications, competencies, and experiences with the test. Any special information or training given to test users prior to their taking the measurements in the study should be described in the test manual.*

> **P18.2.** *Descriptions of where the normative data were obtained must be provided in the test manual.*
> **P18.3.** *Descriptions of the sample studied to obtain the normative data must also be provided.*
> > **P18.3.1.** *Descriptions must be provided in the test manual of how the sample used to obtain the normative data was selected.*
> > **P18.3.2.** *The number of subjects studied to obtain the normative data should be specified in the test manual.*
> > **P18.3.3.** *Evidence must be presented in the test manual to explain how the sample used to obtain normative data is characteristic of the population for whom the measurement is intended to be used.**

All of the requirements described in the previous paragraph relate to whether normative data will be **representative.** A sample should be representative of a population, and the size of the sample should be sufficiently large in order for measurements on a sample to reflect the measurements in the population. The representativeness of the sample relies on the careful construction and application of appropriate operational definitions and sampling methods, topics that go beyond the scope of this *Primer* (the interested reader is urged to consult any of the standard resources on research design that include discussions of sampling).[16,17] Well-designed tests and fully developed tests, however, should have manuals that describe normative data obtained from hundreds or thousands of subjects.

Sometimes, test users will think they are using normative data, when in reality they are basing judgments on criterion referencing. For example, you read an article describing isokinetic quadriceps femoris muscle peak torque measurements in six professional hockey players. The author of the article suggests he has provided "normative data" for professional hockey players. He has not! The sample would be too small, and odds are the standard deviation would be enormous. What has been provided, however, is an insight into what kinds of torque some hockey players attain. You could, if in your professional judgment you thought this was correct, use these values as a goal. In this case, you judge the hockey players to have a torque level that you consider a desirable criterion for your patient.

There is no hard and fast rule as to the size of the sample from which norms should be generated. Some sources suggest that more accurate results are obtained with larger numbers of people tested but only if the sample is representative of the population of interest. Generally, a larger sample will be more representative of a population than will be a smaller sample, but only if the sample is properly drawn. Just how large is large? The advice varies, and the topic is far more complex than can be adequately discussed in this *Primer*.

Because normative data should only be used when they represent the population, the methods used to sample and obtain the data are critical. The *Standards* state:

> **P18.5.** *Descriptions of the methods and research design used to obtain the normative data must be provided in the test manual. Normative data should be obtained using the same measurement procedures that are described in the manual. If other versions of the test were used to obtain the normative data, or if other scales were used, there must be a discussion of how the normative data relate to the data that can be obtained using the test described in the manual.* *

This emphasizes that the measurements used to obtain normative data must have been obtained the same way that we obtain *measurements clinically* if we are to relate our clinical measurements to the normative data.

If you were given, for example, normative data for stride length obtained through use of a sophisticated computer-based motion analysis system, could you use these data with measurements obtained with a stopwatch? A different, but simple and inexpensive, system? The answer is: No! Unless, of course, there are data to show that this simple stopwatch system provides measurements that are interchangeable (equal) with those obtained with the computer-based motion analysis system. Later, we will describe what is required for interchangeability (ie, **parallel-forms reliability**).

Normative data should only be used with measurements similarly obtained. In addition, there may be other limitations on the use of normative data. The *Standards* state:

P18.6. *A complete discussion of limitations in the use of the supplied normative data must be provided in the test manual. The discussion may include, but should not be limited to, considerations of whether the normative data relate to a particular local area, facility, ethnic group, age group, or gender.**

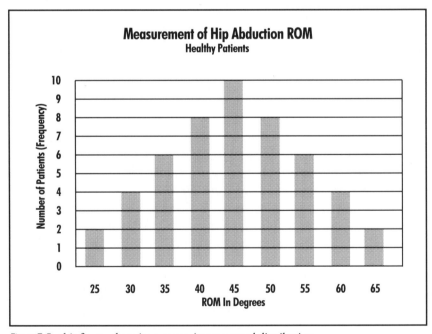

Figure 7. In this figure, there is an approximate normal distribution.

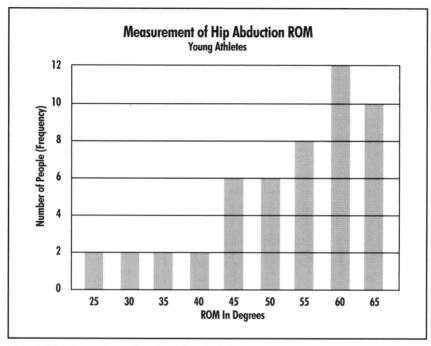

Figure 8. This figure shows data skewed to the left.

Most authorities urge caution in establishing and using norms based on assumptions about whether measurements are normally distributed. For example, the incidence or occurrence of diseases is usually not a phenomenon in which a normal distribution can be assumed. The same caution should apply to any attribute for which normality of a distribution cannot be assumed. When a normal distribution is not present, normative data may actually lead a test user astray in interpreting data. In addition, the use of knowledge about the normal distribution may be misapplied. For example, if someone is ± 2 standard deviations from the mean, that person is among 96% of the population—but that is only true if the measurements are normally distributed. Examine the normal distribution illustrated in Figure 7, and you will see how useful normative data can be. As the figure shows, there is an approximate normal distribution.

Now, consider the problems that might occur if you attempted to interpret measurements obtained from any one of the distributions depicted in Figures 7 through 10, based on your knowledge of the normal distribution.

In Figures 8 and 9, the data are skewed to the left and right, respectively, making use of the standard deviation and normative data problematic. Consider how much worse the problem becomes if the distribution of data is multimodal (ie, has more than one mode), as in the bimodal distribution shown in Figure 10.

How to obtain normative data and how to judge when normative data are good is beyond the scope of the *Primer*.[14] Persons using measurements, however, must consider whether normative data are available and how to use the data whenever they make decisions. The *Standards* place the following obligations on test users:

U3.9. *Test users must understand what constitutes meaningful normative data and how such data can be used.*

U44.3.1.1.*Test users using normative data should interpret any measurement that is interval or ratio scaled in terms of how that measurement relates to measures of central tendency, measures of variability, and percentiles.*

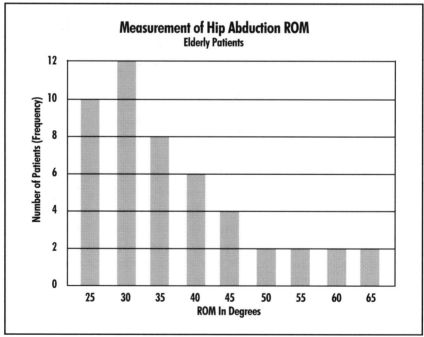

Figure 9. This figure shows data skewed to the right.

U45.10. *Test users, in reports of test results, should relate their measurements to normative data, if available. Test users should report the source of the normative data they use and, if necessary, discuss how applicable the data are to the measurements they are reporting.**

There are guides to determining whether data are normally distributed. **Kurtosis,** which was discussed previously, reflects how peaked or flat a curve is. A normally distributed set of measurements will have a kurtosis of 0. When kurtosis has a positive value, there is a greater-than-normal peak **(leptokurtic),** with the magnitude indicating the extent of the peak. Similarly, when kurtosis has a negative value **(platykurtic),** this indicates a flatter-than-normal curve. The larger the negative number, the flatter the curve.

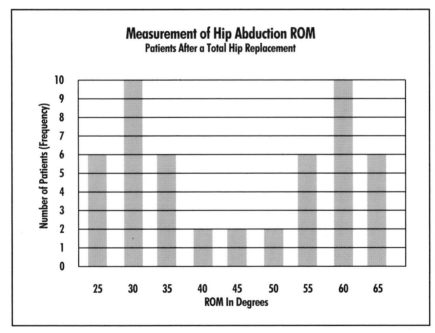

Figure 10. The data in this figure illustrate a bimodal distribution, an example of one type of multimodal distribution.

A second guide to determining whether a distribution deviates from the normal distribution is the **measure of skewedness**. With a perfectly symmetrical normal distribution, the **skewedness index** will be 0. When the distribution is asymmetrical, the skewedness index will have a positive or negative value, indicating the magnitude and direction of the skew.

A variety of mathematical operations exist for transforming scores (eg, Z-transformations, logarithmic transformations). The purpose of many of these transformations is to alter the distribution of measurements. When this occurs, test users should understand the consequences of the transformation that was used to create the norms, as well as the consequences of transforming the measurements obtained.

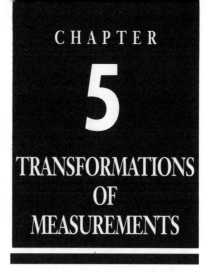

CHAPTER

5

TRANSFORMATIONS
OF
MEASUREMENTS

T he transformation of measurements is not the same thing as the transformation of scales discussed earlier (see page 22). The **transformation of scales,** from a higher form of scale (for example, ratio or interval) to a lower form of scale (for example, ordinal), entails aggregating the numerical values of measurements originally obtained on a quantitative scale into categories on an ordinal scale for the purpose of counting the frequencies of occurrence in the categories. This results in substituting one kind of data or measurement on the original scale for another kind of data or measurement on a different kind of scale.

The **transformation of measurements** consists of doing an arithmetic operation on each numerical value originally obtained. This results in altering the individual numerical values of the measurements. If the transformation of measurements is intended to alter the shape of the distribution to bring it more in line with the normal curve, the transformation that is done is referred to as the **normalization** of the measurements.

Unfortunately, normalization as a method of changing a distribution's characteristics is not the only form of normalization that physical therapists deal with. For example, "normalization" is often used in kinesiological electromyography (EMG) to refer to the quantity of electrical activity, expressed as a percentage of the possible maximum, obtained for a given muscle group in the individual tested. Torque is sometimes expressed as a percentage of body weight. These "normalizations" are not done to change the distribution, but rather *to account for individual differences that could not otherwise be eliminat-*

ed. One could argue that expressing the quantity of anything as a percentage of some agreed-upon, absolute or relative standard quantity is an act of redefining the dimension of interest (the variable), not normalizing the measurements. In any case, what is often called "normalization" (as occurs with kinesiological EMG or torques) is the production of a **derived measurement.** Test users must be very careful to note which type of normalization is being used whenever the term "normalization" appears.

In the *Standards,* **normalization** is defined as

> *... a process that yields a new or transformed measurement that is mathematically derived to change the distribution of measurements; normalization procedures are often used to change the distribution of data to make the distribution more congruent with a bell-shaped (or normal) curve.**

When measurements are transformed, the person who does the transforming should have sound theoretical reasons for doing so and should convey a clear sense of the dimension or attribute that underlies the transformed measurements; that is, the transformed measurements should be measurements of something that has to do with the original dimension or attribute.

The **transformation of measurements** is defined in the *Standards* as

> *... the application of a mathematical operation for the purpose of changing the value or distribution of measurements, such as is done in the processes of standardization or normalization.**

Standardization is also one of those words that has two distinct meanings. The *Standards* define **standardization** as

> *... a process by which a score is converted (transformed) into a relative score by using indices of central tendency and variability; a commonly used standardized score is the z score.**

The term "standardization" is also used to describe the process of systematization (standardizing) of the methods used to obtain a measurement. Standardization of methods, however, does not ensure reliability, because reliability can only be determined through the collection of data. Once again, caution must be exercised so that the proper use of the word and method occurs.

The transformation of measurements arose initially in psychology and education. In educational and psychological testing, the desire to compare the performance of one individual with another of his same age group or class group, and the desire to compare the performance of an individual on one kind of test (eg, English) with his or her performance on another kind of test (eg, mathematics), gave rise to the notion of **standard measures** and **standard scores**.

A standard measure *(which is a simplified version of a standardized score)* is an individual measurement in a set of measurements expressed in terms of the number of standard deviations it deviates from—either above or below—the mean of the set of measurements. Operationally, a standard measure (frequently referred to as a *z* **score**) is obtained by subtracting the mean from the individual measurement and then dividing the remainder by the standard deviation. A standard measure (a *z* score) may be either positive or negative and may vary in size. Turning individual measurements into standard measures does not alter the distribution of the original measurements. By definition, the mean of a set of standard measures is zero and the standard deviation is 1.0.

The dimension of interest in standard measures is the number of standard deviations above or below the mean. Standard measures have a unique usefulness in enabling one to say that Johnny is better in Algebra than in English and Social Studies because he is 2 standard deviations above the mean in Algebra and just 1 standard deviation above the mean in the other two subjects. Standard measures are one step removed from indicating the quantity of the attribute tested, but they are not so abstract as to render the idea useless in physical therapy. Standard measures might be useful in comparing measurements obtained on individuals, in much the same manner as the original idea in psychology and education. The usefulness of standard measures, however, remains to be demonstrated and popularized in physical therapy.

One potential use of standard measures is in the examination of gait. There are many variables that can be measured in gait. If we wanted to know, for example, how walking speed compared with stride length, we could use standard measures and find that in one case a person's measurements were higher than the mean and in the other case lower. We could also identify how the person's measurements compared on two very different variables with those obtained from other persons (eg, speed was 1 standard deviation above the mean, and stride length was 0.75 standard deviation below the mean).

Transforming measurements for the purpose of **normalizing the distribution** of the measurements can be a complicated operation. The reasons underlying the transformation of measurements have to do principally with concerns for practicality and convenience. There should also be a sound theoretical basis for the transformation, and the consequences of the transformation need to be fully understood.

Persons who develop, sell, or promote the use of tests should provide, as stated in the *Standards* (P18.7), "... details on any data transformations (eg, any standardization or normalization procedures) used in obtaining or preparing the normative data."* Similarly, the *Standards* state:

> **U45.11** *Test users reporting the results of their tests should indicate whether any data were transformed (normalized or standardized). Test users, in their reports, should justify the use of transformations, if this is not customary practice.*

Whether measurements are normalized in order to change a distribution or to eliminate some individual differences, as was the case with the kinesiological EMG example, test users must take into account the effect of the process on the measurement. If a test user wants to relate to normative data or even to any other data, the test user must have data in the same form as the normalized data being used for comparison. For example, researchers often normalize force measurements as a percentage of a person's maximal isometric force production or as a percentage of the person's body weight. The measurements they report, and the phenomena they then describe, will only exist in clinical practice if the measurements obtained in clinical practice are similarly obtained (ie, if the measurements are expressed as a percentage of maximal isometric force or body weight). Such normalizations are often impractical in the clinical setting. The process also is not only time consuming, but it may potentially introduce more error into the measurement because multiple measurements must be obtained.

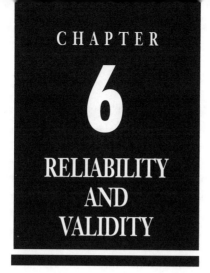

Introductory Comments and Concepts

T he **reliability** and **validity** of a measurement have to do with the trust-worthiness of a measurement, that is, the confidence that can be placed in a measurement. Is the measurement *reproducible*, and does it provide *meaningful* information? Not all measurement techniques yield equally useful data. For example, do you always agree with your colleague about MMT grades above Fair? This is an issue of reliability. Or can you predict with some certainty from some measurements of muscle force production that an athlete can return to competition? This is an issue of validity.

Reliability and validity are related but have different characteristics. A measurement cannot be valid (meaningful) if it is not reliable (reproducible), but a reliable measurement is not necessarily a valid measurement. Without reliability, there can be no validity, but reliability alone does not ensure validity.

Think of this example from outside the physical therapy field. Some people claim that measurements of "personality" can be obtained from analyzing handwriting samples. This is a claim for the validity of handwriting analyses in producing authentic and believable, and therefore useful, measurements of personality. When we refer to usefulness of the analysis, we ask whether these handwriting measurements of personality could be trusted when selecting people to be spouses, co-workers, students, patients, physicians, holders of political office, and so forth. For the claim to be correct, two different handwriting analysts using the same method of analysis, or one handwriting analyst using a single method on two different occasions, should never come to strongly **dissimilar (unreliable)** measurements of "personality."

Without reliability, there can be no validity. But suppose, on the other hand, that the measurements are in fact reliable. They are reliable because **identical (perfectly reliable)** measurements of "personality" are obtained on handwriting samples by two different handwriting analysts using the same method of handwriting analysis. Or they may be reliable because one analyst using the same method on two different occasions came to the same conclusion. The measurements of "personality" may be perfectly reliable, yet incorrect or unbelievable **(invalid)**. Reliability, therefore, does not ensure validity, and without validity, a measurement has little value.

Issues related to reliability and validity can be quite complex. Fortunately, there is a vast body of knowledge on these topics, albeit not necessarily related to physical therapy measurements. Test users (clinicians) are obligated to understand reliability and validity because, without such understanding, tests cannot be used properly and measurements are really uninterpretable.

Reliability refers to the reproducibility or repeatability of measurements. There are, however, many forms of reliability, and each has its own definition. The following definitions are from the *Standards*:

> *Reliability: the consistency or repeatability of measurements; the degree to which measurements are error-free and the degree to which repeated measurements will agree.*
>
> *Intratester reliability: the consistency or equivalence of measurements when one person takes repeated measurements separated in time; indicates agreement in measurements over time.*
>
> *Test-retest reliability: the consistency of repeated measurements separated in time; indicates stability (reliability) over time.*
>
> *Intertester reliability: the consistency or equivalence of measurements when more than one person takes the measurements; indicates agreement of measurements taken by different examiners.*
>
> *Parallel-forms (alternate-forms) reliability: the consistency or agreement of measurements obtained with different (alternative) forms of a test; indicates whether measurements obtained with different forms of a test can be used interchangeably.*
>
> *Internal consistency: the extent to which items or elements that contribute to a measurement reflect one basic phenomenon or dimension.**

Some people say a measurement is valid if the measurement reflects what it is supposed to reflect. This, however, is an inadequate definition. A more useful definition is that validity has to do with whether measurements can be used for the purpose(s) for which they are intended. Validity has to do with the uses to which measurements are put. Valid measurements are authentic or believable in the sense that they can be used for the purpose(s) for which they are intended. A measurement can be valid for one purpose, but not another. A grade on an anatomy examination may be a valid indicator of knowledge of anatomy, but it does not necessarily indicate whether someone is intelligent, knows something about physiology, or is able to use that knowledge of anatomy in a kinesiology course.

Validity deals with specified uses of a measurement. There are many forms of validity, and each has its own definition. The following definitions are from the *Standards*:

Validity: the degree to which a useful (meaningful) interpretation can be inferred from a measurement.

Construct validity: the conceptual (theoretical) basis for using a measurement to make an inferred interpretation; evidence for construct validity is through logical argumentation based on theoretical and research evidence.

Content validity: a form of validity that deals with the extent to which a measurement is judged to reflect the meaningful elements of a construct and not any extraneous elements.

Criterion-based (criterion-related) validity: three forms of criterion-based validity exist: concurrent validity, predictive validity, and prescriptive validity; the common element is that, with each of these forms of validity, the correctness of an inferred interpretation can be tested by comparing a measurement with either a different measurement or data obtained by other forms of testing.

Concurrent validity: a form of criterion-based validity in which an inferred interpretation is justified by comparing a measurement with supporting evidence that was obtained at approximately the same time as the measurement being validated.

Predictive validity: a form of criterion-based validity in which an inferred interpretation is justified by comparing a measurement with sup-

porting evidence that is obtained at a later point in time; examines the justification of using a measurement to say something about future events or conditions.

Prescriptive validity: *a form of criterion-based validity in which the inferred interpretation of a measurement is the determination of the form of treatment a person is to receive; prescriptive validity is justified based on the successful outcome of the chosen treatment.**

Validity

Construct Validity

Before a measurement can be obtained, you must have an idea about what you want to quantify or characterize. You would have to know that hitting a tendon causes a reflex response before you could develop a test of deep tendon reflexes. In addition, unless you knew that reflexes were either exaggerated or diminished with pathology, you would be unable to develop meaningful categories for the classification of reflex responses. In this example, knowledge of reflexes, the nervous system, and neuropathology provides the theoretical basis for the development of a testing procedure (the use of a reflex hammer) and a measurement (the reflex response). This knowledge, this theoretical underpinning, is the **construct** upon which the test and measurement are developed. Construct validity is demonstrated through logical presentation of information that supports the procedures used in the test and the usefulness of the obtained measurements. There is no simple, absolute, direct test of construct validity; rather, evidence is brought to bear from a variety of sources. Research evidence can add to the argument for construct validity, but it can never directly or absolutely test the correctness of a construct.

Content Validity

Almost all people who have been students understand the issues related to content validity. An anatomy test on the upper extremity would certainly be expected to have questions on the course of the radial nerve and the muscles innervated by that nerve. If you took a test that never asked a single question about that nerve or the muscles innervated by the nerve, the test would be incomplete. Any grade obtained on the test would not accurately reflect a person's knowledge of the upper extremity. The test score (a measurement) would lack validity, because the test did not adequately sample the relevant elements (**content**) of the attribute (knowledge of the upper extremity) being measured.

Issues of content validity are major obstacles in the development of functional assessments, work screening measurements, and even tests of muscle performance. In each of these cases, we have little evidence to suggest how many different elements must be tested in order to have a meaningful measurement. For example, what tests should be used to contribute to a measurement of readiness to return to work after low back injury?

Content validity is strongly linked to construct validity. In order to know what elements must be considered for testing, there must be a theoretical basis for a measurement. For example, we needed an operational definition of the upper extremity before we could even entertain the question as to whether our test adequately covered all the material it should.

Content validity, like construct validity, can never be directly and absolutely tested. Evidence that suggests what elements should be reflected in a measurement is brought to bear from a variety of sources. Research evidence can add to the argument for content validity, but it can never directly or absolutely test whether all relevant elements are reflected in the measurement.

Criterion-based (Criterion-related) Validity

Validity deals with the usefulness of a measurement (ie, what inferences can be made). A theoretical basis (a construct) for the test makes it more likely to have meaning, as does an adequate sample of relevant items (content validity). But, the critical issue is whether the measurement can really be put to use. Does a measurement of intelligence tell us whether a person can really solve problems? Do muscle tests really reflect a person's functional capacity? Do developmental tests really reflect maturation of the nervous system?

The various forms of criterion-based validity examine whether a measurement can be put to specific use. In each case, a test of validity can, when possible, be obtained by comparing the measurement being examined with another measurement or a series of other measurements. The criterion measurement (the one being used for comparison) should have a known level of usefulness. We validate a measurement of unknown validity by comparing it with another measurement (a criterion) of known validity. An obvious problem arises when you are the first to attempt to measure something. What standard do you use for comparison? In practice, multiple tests, including measurements that reflect similar attributes, may be used as the criteria.

If, for example, we were developing a balance test for persons with hemiplegia and no similar test previously existed, how could we show the validity for our categorizations of good balance, moderate balance, or poor balance? We could use the following to demonstrate criterion-based validity: We could see how often persons in each of our categories fell, we could measure how long persons in each of our categories were able to perform functional activities while standing, or we could ask family members how often the patients needed to grab for support at home.

Demonstrating criterion-related validity for new measurements may seem like an impossible task, but, as our example illustrated, with some effort and creativity, evidence for or against criterion validity can be accumulated. The nature of the evidence, however, will differ depending on the type of criterion-related validity being examined. Each type of criterion-related validity relates to how a measurement is used.

Although all forms of criterion-related validity can have evidence brought to bear directly showing validity or a lack of validity, there is a danger in thinking of a measurement as being either valid or invalid. Almost all measurements contain some information; the more valid the measurement, the more useful the information. *Validity is not an all-or-none proposition.* Test users need to know how much confidence they can place in inferences based on measurements. Test users, therefore, must know about the validity of their measurements and appreciate the subtlety of the arguments for and against use of the measurements. A measurement has some degree of validity and should never be classified as being valid or invalid. A measurement can only be valid for a specified purpose.

Concurrent Validity

Sometimes, we use a measurement to make a judgment about how something is at the present time. When we want to infer something about phenomena at the time the measurements were obtained, we need to show concurrent validity for our measurements. The hypothetical balance test we proposed would yield such measurements. Our measurements were supposed to tell us how good each patient's balance was at the time the patient took the test.

Manual muscle test grades are often used to make inferences about a patient's status at the time the test is given. One inference is whether a muscle is innervated (the original purpose of MMT as developed by Lovett).[18] We could provide evidence for concurrent validity of the inference relating to innervation by comparing MMT grades, particularly those below Fair, with the results of electrodiagnostic testing. If we collected a sizable amount of data showing a relationship between MMT grades and electrodiagnostic test results, we could say that we have provided evidence for the concurrent validity of MMT grades as indicators of innervation status.

If, however, we then wanted to use MMT grades to infer whether a person could ambulate, we would need to establish concurrent validity for this use (inference). This demonstrates that every specific use of a measurement must be subjected to examination for all the appropriate types of validity. Even the theoretical bases (constructs) for using MMT grades to indicate innervation status and functional status are vastly different. This example demonstrates that measurements can only be valid for a stated purpose. It is inappropriate to state that a measurement is valid unless the specific use of the measurement is described and it is even more inappropriate to state that a test or a device has been shown to be valid. Tests and devices may yield measurements that are useful (valid), but the tests and devices themselves cannot be valid. *Validity, like reliability, is a property of a measurement, not a property of a test or a device.*

Predictive Validity

Often, we measure in order to make predictions about the future. When we check the treads on our car tires, we not only want to know how much wear has occurred (a concurrent judgment), we also often want to estimate how much longer the tires will last (a predictive judgment). In order for us to make predictions, we need to have some evidence that measurements lead to predictions that come true. Such evidence supports the **predictive validity** of a measurement. This is a very important form of validity, because all screening tests are based on predictive validity. Screening is based on the assumption that after detecting something, we can intervene and alter what would otherwise occur. Unless the measurement really predicts a future event, how can we know whether the intervention was useful or necessary? Predictive validity is a prerequisite for any screening test.

Employment screening tests, particularly those that test low back function, can only be justified if the measurements they yield have been shown to have predictive validity. When persons are tested as a condition of employment or they are tested as a condition for returning to work, the measurement is being used to predict whether the person might be hurt on the job. But how do we know that the person really would be injured?

Predictive validity is demonstrated by obtaining measurements and then observing whether predictions based on the measurement come true. Unfortunately, we often become so convinced that our predictions will come true that we feel it is impossible not to intervene and, therefore, we cannot test whether the measurements are predictive. This is often the case with some low back testing and employment screening, as well as with postural screening programs and preseason athletic testing. Because of our frequent inability to refrain from interventions, we can see the importance of collecting data on the predictive validity of a measurement before the use of that measurement becomes so popular that scientific testing becomes difficult.

Prescriptive Validity

Each type of criterion-related validity deals with a different type of use for a measurement. A measurement with concurrent validity allows us to make some inference about what is occurring at the time the measurement was taken. A measurement with predictive validity allows us to say something about future events or the future status of something. **Prescriptive validity** is very similar to predictive validity, but a measurement with prescriptive validity guides us in providing an intervention. If a person tests positive for the human immunodeficiency virus (HIV), this indicates the presence of the acquired immunodeficiency syndrome (AIDS) virus, and more importantly that at present there is essentially a 100% chance that the person will develop AIDS at some future date. A variety of experimental methods are being used to delay or prevent the onset of the disease, but at present the measurement (the classification of HIV positive or negative) provides no guidance as to which intervention should be used. Testing for HIV has predictive validity for the appearance of AIDS, but no prescriptive validity. If the measurement allowed a determination of which variant of the virus was present and then provided guidance as to which intervention to choose, the measurement would also have prescriptive validity.

If, for example, the purpose of a wheelchair is to prevent deformities in a child with cerebral palsy, we could use a measurement to determine which type of wheelchair should be used. Proving prescriptive validity for this measurement would be simple. If measurements were obtained on a large number of children and, based on these measurements, different wheelchairs were prescribed for different children, we would need to know whether the deformities were prevented. We would be especially interested in knowing whether there was a lower incidence of deformities when the wheelchairs were chosen based on the measurement as compared with when chairs were chosen based on other criteria.

Prescriptive validity has a role whenever someone suggests a test or a series of tests can yield measurements that lead to a choice of treatments. Evidence for the prescriptive validity of a measurement comes in the form of data that demonstrate that the treatment was effective. This is because the purpose of the measurement was to guide treatment choice. Therefore, if the treatment accomplished nothing, the measurement would have no prescriptive value.

Issues Related to Validity

Norm Referencing and Criterion Referencing

Because validity deals with the usefulness (the inferential capacity) of measurements, we need to consider how measurements are used to make judgments. In this *Primer*, we have previously described the normal distribution and how judgments can be made by comparing a single measurement with those obtained from other members of a population. These types of judgments are said to be based on **norm referencing**. This simply means a judgment is made not based on how good or bad or how big or small a measurement is, but rather solely on how the measurement relates to measurements taken from a representative sample of the population.

Norm referencing is very different from another type of judgment call, **criterion referencing**. Inferences from measurements are often made based on whether we believe the values mean something. When we examine a patient and state that the patient's posture is poor, we are **criterion referencing** because we are making a judgment based on a standard that we believe represents an ideal or an acceptable model. This must be the case, because there are no normative data for postural alignment!

When we make a judgment based on norm referencing, the inference is clear: If a person is different from his or her peers, then that means something. What it means, however, is not always clear. How much deviation indicates that there is a problem? With criterion referencing, there is an even bigger problem. On what basis did we establish the criterion? Who, for example, came up with the idea that 70% on an examination in school was the criterion for acceptable (passing) test performance? Where is the evidence that someone who gets a 70% (C) in a course knows an acceptable amount of knowledge, whereas someone with a 69% or less must take a course over (presuming, of course, that a D was unacceptable to that person)? Similarly, we might ask: Where did our current concepts (criteria) for acceptable postural alignment, relative to a plumb line, come from? How do we know this alignment is good, ideal, or even desirable?

Judgments based on norm referencing and criterion referencing are of specific types. They may lead to judgments about concurrent phenomena, future phenomena, or actions that need to be taken. Decisions based on comparisons with a standard (criterion referencing) or comparisons with a population (norm referencing) must still be validated in the context of the appropriate type of validity (eg, concurrent, predictive, or prescriptive).

Indices Used to Assess the Validity of Measurements

A variety of indices are available that can be used to evaluate how much information is contained in a measurement. For measurements that are categorical judgments about the presence or absence of a disease or some other attribute, there are many indices. The following section provides definitions and discusses the implications of these indices.

False classifications. When something is judged to be present or absent, there are two types of errors that can be made. **False negatives** occur when someone is classified as not having some attribute, even though that person really has the attribute. **False positives** occur when someone tests positively for some attribute but in fact does not have that attribute. In either case, a measurement would be in error, and there would be no validity for the measurement. In practice, false negatives and false positives are calculated as a percentage of a group that has been tested for some attribute. A percentage for false positives and false negatives is then calculated and can be used to interpret subsequent observations.

If you knew that there is an 80% false negative rate when a disease is said to be present, there would be little solace in a negative classification, because 80% of those told they do not have the disease would in fact be sick! Not only would the results provide little comfort, you might even choose to take medicine for the disease although the test indicated you did not have the disease.

Because almost everyone past the age of 30 years shows arthritic changes in the vertebrae of their cervical spines,[19] one could argue that anyone who made a diagnosis of symptomatic arthritis based on radiographs would have a remarkably large number of false positives. Consider the implications if people were given treatment based solely on radiographic findings.

False negative rates and false positive rates are nonprobabilistic estimates of error. They show the error associated with a number of tests but do not provide probabilistic estimates of what would occur under other uses of the same test. The rates of false positives and false negatives describe what is found in the sample studied and are not adjusted to make more accurate predictions about what might be found when other samples are examined.

True classifications. Just as there may be errors when determining the absence of any attribute, so may there be errors when finding that something is present. True negatives occur when a negative finding is made for some attribute and the attribute is not present. A true positive occurs when a person tests positively for some attribute actually present. The issues with true classifications are the same as those for false classifications. The difference, however, is that the higher the percentage of true classifications that can be made, the more valid and useful the classifications.

Predictive value of a measurement. Classifications about the presence or absence of a diagnostic finding might appear to carry equal information, but that is not the case. For some measurements made on some groups of people, a negative finding may carry a greater level of certainty (more information) than would a positive finding. For other measurements made on other groups, a positive finding may carry more information. Negative or positive findings can only be partially understood by looking at false positive and false negative rates. The **predictive values** of a measurement tell us far more about what we can use a classification for, and with what certainty.

The predictive value indicates the degree of certainty that can be associated with a positive or negative finding (measurement) obtained by use of a diagnostic test. The **predictive value of a positive measurement** is the ratio formed by dividing the number of true positives by all positive findings. The **predictive value of a negative measurement** is the ratio formed by dividing the number of true negatives by the number of all negative findings.

For example, Sinacore and Ehsani[20] illustrated this concept by creating the following hypothetical example. In 100 persons who reported atypical chest pain there were 50 known to have coronary artery disease (CAD) and 50 who did not have CAD. Based on an exercise test, it was found that among the 50 without CAD, there were 45 true negatives and 5 false positives. Among those with CAD, there were 32 true positives and 18 false negatives. *The predictive value of the positive classification was*

Predictive Value of a Positive Test = True Positives/(True Positives + False Positives)
Predictive Value of a Positive Test = 32/(32+5)= .86

The predictive value of a negative classification was

Predictive Value of a NegativeTest = True Negatives/(True Negatives + False Negatives)
Predictive Value of a Negative Test = 45/(45+18)= .71

From the values calculated, it is clear that a positive classification carries more certainty than a negative classification. Persons with a positive finding can be more certain that they have the disease than can persons who have a negative finding be certain that they do not have the disease. In other words, many persons who would appear to be disease-free (100%-71%=29%) may have the disease, whereas only 14% (100%-86%) of those who believe they have the disease would be falsely concerned. This latter number, though smaller than the predictive value of the negative test, could be quite consequential. If the predictive value of a positive classification is low, then the possibility of excessive management, including unnecessary treatments, medications, and even surgeries, is possible. This can be contrasted to what occurs when the predictive value of a negative finding is low and persons who may have the disease are not given treatment.

Sensitivity and specificity of a classification. Another way of evaluating whether we have made correct judgments based on the presence or absence of a diagnostic finding is to consider the sensitivity and specificity of a test. **Sensitivity of a classification** is an indication of how well a diagnostic test identifies people who *should have a positive finding*. The sensitivity is calculated by forming a ratio from the number of persons with a true positive response on a test and dividing this number by the number of persons who should have had a positive response (ie, the number of persons who are known to have properties that would indicate that they should test positive). A **sensitive test** (one with a high ratio) is one that finds something when it should. A test with **low sensitivity** often fails to find something when it should. We might wonder what the sensitivity is for classifications used by physical therapists. Are tests that lead to classifications of hypermobility or hypomobility of lumbar segments sensitive? Are tests for muscle tightness or stretch weakness sensitive?

Sometimes the issue is whether a classification correctly identifies those who do not have some attribute. If a sensitive test finds something when it is present, then an index is needed to show how well a test does in showing the absence of something (a negative finding) when it is not present. The **specificity of a measurement (classification)** is an indication of how well a diagnostic test identifies people who *should have a negative finding*. The specificity is calculated by forming a ratio of the number of persons with a true negative response on a test and dividing this number by the number of persons who should have had a negative response (ie, the number of persons should test negative).

In physical therapy practice, we sometimes have findings that are so ubiquitous that we have to wonder what they mean. For example, almost everyone has some postural anomaly. In a person with musculoskeletal pain, is it diagnostic to observe a forward head, excessive lordosis, or unequal shoulder heights? Or, does the commonplace nature of these findings suggest that tests for these anomalies may have little specificity (ie, while they may indicate a postural fault, they do not indicate a postural fault related to the patient's symptoms)?

We can also illustrate sensitivity and specificity by using Sinacore and Ehsani's example.[18] *The sensitivity of a classification is*

Sensitivity = Number of Persons With True Positives/Number of Persons Who Should Be Positive
Sensitivity = 32/50= .64, .64x100=64%

The specificity of the classification is

Specificity = Number of Persons With True Negatives/Number of Persons Who Should Be Negative
Specificity = 45/50= .90, .90x100=90%

In these examples, the sensitivity of the classification is only 64%. Many people (100%-64%=36%) with the disease who should have a positive classification are missed. On the other hand, few people (100%-90%=10%) who should have a negative finding are falsely identified as having the disease because of the high specificity (90%). Few persons (10%) who do not have the disease would get treatment because of the high specificity; unfortunately, many persons (36%) with the disease would also not get treatment because of the low sensitivity.

Judging Validity

Creators of tests can make a case that their tests yield measurements that may be valid for a given purpose. Criterion-related validity requires that a measurement be compared with a measurement of known validity. We are comparing the unknown inferential use of one measurement against the known inferential use of another measurement. There are many kinds of research in which this is done, but often there is no simple singular comparison possible. For example, if there is no measurement that reflects whether a person can return to work, how do we validate a recently developed work-screening measurement? We must use multiple sources and various kinds of data to test the correctness of our inference. We might, for example, find that our measurement relates to the amount of disability payments in the year after screening and to some extent to the days a person lost from work. In an attempt to validate the use of a measurement, we often compile evidence, even when it comes to criterion-based validity. Ideally, when we examine criterion-based validity, we would like to compare a measurement against another measurement, but that is not always possible.

An additional concern about judging validity, even when we can make simple comparisons, is the reality that no measurement is perfect or always has perfect inferential capacity. A measurement is valid for a use to some extent and will always have some error associated with it. Assessments of false positives and negatives, predictive values of tests, and specificity and sensitivity are all attempts to assess the degree of validity associated with tests used to classify. Correlation coefficients and other statistical indices are used to indicate to what extent inferences may be correct. *A measurement is not valid or invalid; rather, a measurement has some degree of validity for a specified purpose.* We use research literature to gain insight into the degree of validity and the purpose and the evidence available for each claim.

Sometimes, we simply do not have data to demonstrate the validity of an inference we want to make from a measurement. Clinical practice often requires that we must make judgments and decisions before research data are available. In these cases, however, the need for validity still exists, even as we proceed in the absence of evidence. The *Standards* suggest:

U3.2. *Test users must understand the differences between clinical opinions (impressions) that are not based on valid measurements and inferences that are based on the use of valid measurements.**

In addition, the *Standards* note that a test user should always note in the clinical documentation when an observation is based on the validated use of a measurement or on a clinical impression.

Reliability

Any quantitative measurement really consists of two components; one reflects what is being measured, and the other is made up of error. Therefore:

Measurement = True Measurement + Measurement Error

When we assess reliability, we are determining how much of the measurement is true measurement and how much is error. When we assess the reliability of categorical measurements, we are determining whether errors occurred when we made assignments to categories. Because we never really know what part of the measurement represents the true measurement, we examine reliability by considering the stability or agreement between different sets of measurements. Measurements that can be repeated may not actually represent true measurements, but they are more likely to represent true measurements than those that vary for unaccountable reasons.

Reliability deals with the stability (consistency) of a measurement. This seems to contradict what we use measurements for, because often we measure things to determine whether changes are taking place. A measurement should, however, reflect only the attribute that is being described or quantified. When the attribute changes, the measurement should change, but other factors may account for changes in the measurements. We may assume that MMT grades are supposed to reflect the ability of a patient's muscle to generate forces. Many factors that have nothing to do with the variable we are trying to measure, however, may make these grades vary. For example, if a patient has just had surgery, the MMT grade may reflect how the anesthesia is affecting the patient and not what the muscle is actually capable of achieving. Similarly, MMT grades of a depressed person may reflect the person's psychological state rather than a physiologic state.

If a measurement is to convey useful information (ie, have some level of validity), it should not vary when there is no change in what is being measured. Reliability must be present to some extent if there is to be any level of validity. A measurement, however, may be quite stable (ie, reliable) but convey no meaningful information, and therefore have little or no validity. Sometimes people will refer to random and nonrandom errors affecting the reliability of measurements. From a practical standpoint, any error that cannot be accounted for in a measurement interferes with the usefulness of a measurement. Random errors certainly cannot be accounted for in the interpretation of measurements. Systematic errors, however, that have not been identified also cannot be accounted for in the interpretation of measurements. If we know, for example, that all second measurements of ROM increased by a given amount (a form of systematic error), we could interpret all second measurements accordingly. If, however, there was such an increase and we did not know it existed, then we would mistakenly believe that ROM was increasing when the increase was a function of our taking measurements a second time (ie, a problem with reliability).

There are three basic sources of unwanted variability in measurements that lessen reliability: lability in what is being measured, errors in the test or instrument, and errors by the person taking the measurement. When measurement variability occurs due to any of these factors and this error can be eliminated mathematically, then this is no longer a source of error.

The source of error that is hardest to comprehend relates to lability of the measurement. Excessive lability occurs when variables are influenced by so many factors that we cannot account for or control these factors and as a result the measurement fluctuates to an unacceptable degree without identifiable causes.

Sometimes, we attempt to measure things that are so changeable that we are unlikely to get good information. *If the attribute we are measuring is very labile, we may never get a reliable measurement.* A postural assessment of a patient with athetosis would make no sense, but what about gait measurements of a patient with ataxia? Often, the characteristics that contribute to the lability of the measurement may be transient. For example, a patient awaking from a night's sleep may find instructions hard to follow and perform poorly on a test of coordination. The patient would exhibit lability. The same patient, however, tested when more widely awake may not exhibit that degree of lability. Test users must be aware of factors that could influence measurements aside from changes in the variable of interest.

The second source of error is the test or the procedures. *The test (including any instruments) used to obtain the measurements may have a flaw.* This might be as simple as having a plastic goniometer with an offset axis, or as complicated as having a faulty computer attached to a pulmonary function testing device. A questionnaire with an ambiguous question can be thought of as a faulty instrument that might lead to lessened reliability. A fundamentally flawed operational definition could also be a source of instrument error.

The third and most obvious source of poor reliability would be when the person taking the measurement does something wrong. If instructions are inconsistently given to patients, different measurements may be obtained, even though the attribute never changed. Allowing a person with low back pain to relax before attempting a straight-leg-raising test might result in a different measurement than would occur if a therapist simply grabbed a patient's leg and started lifting without any preliminary dialogue. A more subtle error may occur if two therapists testing a patient's ADL allowed different time periods before declaring that the patient could not do some task. Not all examiner errors are necessarily very dramatic. In the real world of measurement, subtle changes in examiner behavior may contribute to variations in measurements. Test users should therefore be wary about deviating from accepted test procedures.

Each form of reliability assesses a different quality of a measurement. Depending on how measurements are used, the different forms of reliability become more or less important. If, for example, different therapists often obtain a measurement from the same patient, then intertester reliability becomes very important. If different forms of a test are used to obtain one type of measurement, then parallel-forms reliability becomes very important.

Intratester Reliability

Intratester reliability represents the consistency of measurements when one person takes repeated measurements separated in time. This indicates stability (reliability) over time. At a bare minimum, it would seem only reasonable that if someone measures something multiple times and there has been no change, the measurements should be very close, if not identical.

Although research has shown that therapists can replicate their own goniometric PROM measurements at most joints,[21] the same may not be true for other measurements. If we are assessing a patient's reflexes (whether the patient is hypotonic or hypertonic), can we replicate the results of our tests, or do we find this phenomenon highly variable? If we see variations and cannot account for these variations, then how can we interpret our measurements? Here, we see how poor intratester reliability may threaten validity.

The very name **intra**tester reliability implies that we are examining whether a single person can obtain measurements that do not vary when the phenomenon being measured has not changed. Intratester reliability, however, demonstrates more than whether a person can replicate a measurement. Because reliability is a property of a measurement, in order for a measurement to be reliable, it must not change in ways that we cannot discern. Therefore, when we examine intratester reliability, we reflect not only on the capacity of the tester to obtain the measurement, we also reflect on the measurement instrument and the stability of what is being measured.

Stability is a particularly important part of intratester reliability. When we examine intratester reliability, it is customary to have one examiner take measurements of the same person or thing on different occasions. We then see whether these sets of measurements agree with each other. Measurements are therefore taken on at least two occasions. If intratester reliability is to be present, the attribute we are measuring should not change in an unpredictable fashion between measurement sessions. A labile measurement may change; a stable measurement would not change.

Not all phenomena remain stable over long periods of time. Certainly, a person with limited knee motion due to an effusion can expect ROM to change over time because of resolution of the swelling. Treatments might also effect a change in ROM because they influenced swelling or some other factor affecting motion. We do not expect measurements to stay the same when there is changing pathology or when interventions are used. We do, however, expect all measurements to have some degree of stability when there is no change in pathology and there is no intervention; otherwise, it would be impossible to use measurements to reflect changes due to altered pathology or intervention. In examining intratester reliability, the test-retest interval has to be chosen with all these issues in mind. The interval should not be so long that changes can be expected in the measurement due to identifiable factors such as aging, disease resolution, and so forth. The interval should also not be artificially brief, but rather should reflect the kind of interval that normally occurs between repeated measurements.

In practice, we find that the test-retest interval for reliability studies is chosen based on many factors, including the practicality of measuring patients more than once. There are no absolute rules or guidelines as to how long the test-retest interval should be. Persons reporting reliability studies should, however, discuss the intervals they used and the implications of these time periods.

Intratester reliability estimates reflect many sources of error. But, they will always indicate how well persons can repeat their own measurements, and to some extent, depending on the test-retest interval, these estimates will also reflect the stability of the measurements. Intratester reliability indicates whether persons can repeatedly obtain the same measurements. Because this form of reliability indicates testers can replicate their own findings, it is desirable. If only this form of reliability is present, however, the measurement will have very limited use. Unless multiple examiners can agree on measurements (intertester reliability), measurements cannot be used in a generalizable fashion; that is, we cannot share information in a meaningful fashion. For example, if two therapists always differed on shoulder-flexion ROM measurements, how would we know who was correct? There is no possibility that measurements from both could validly reflect the motion. This once again illustrates the relationship between reliability and validity.

Intertester Reliability

Intertester reliability reflects the extent to which measurements taken by different examiners agree. We previously noted that measurements are made up of two parts: true measurement and measurement error. To the extent that a measurement is error-free, all persons who take that measurement or make a categorization should agree. A perfectly reliable measurement would be error-free, and all persons who obtain that measurement on the same person would obtain the same value. No measurement is perfect; therefore, persons attempting to take the same measurement often differ by varying amounts.

Consider the following example. Two therapists assessing the same patient each classify the patient differently in terms of the patient's sitting balance. One therapist says the patient has good balance, and the other says the patient has poor balance. Not only does this represent a problem of intertester reliability (ie, there is none), it must be obvious that both cannot correctly reflect the patient's sitting balance—that is, both measurements cannot be valid.

The example demonstrates two important reasons why intertester reliability is important. When therapists cannot replicate each other's measurements, then measurements cannot be used interchangeably. In view of our therapists' inability to agree on a classification of sitting balance, it would be inappropriate to have these two therapists ever evaluate the sitting balance of a patient at different times. The differences in their categorizations could not be interpreted. We would not know whether the change in the categorization was due to a change in sitting balance or simply to the fact that the two therapists classify differently. There must be a reasonable amount of agreement for intertester reliability before anyone can ever justify allowing different persons to measure the same phenomenon at different times.

Our example also demonstrates the second critical reason why we must always be concerned about intertester reliability. Because two therapists assessed the same sitting balance and came up with diverse classifications, we noted that both of their measurements could not be valid; that is, they both could not correctly reflect sitting balance. At best, one of the two therapists was correct, and at worst, they both misrepresented the patient's actual sitting balance. When measurers disagree, validity cannot be universal. When intertester reliability is poor, those obtaining measurements cannot possibly claim the same degree of validity.

Intertester reliability also relates to the terms "subjective" and "objective." The following are the definitions from the *Standards*:

> **Subjective measurement:** *a measurement that is affected by some aspect of the person obtaining the measurement (contrasts with **objective measurement**); subjectivity relates to the reliability of measurements, especially the intertester reliability; the more subjective the measurement, the less reliable is the measurement; subjectivity, like reliability, is measured along a continuum.*

Objective measurement: a measurement that is not affected by some aspect of the person obtaining the measurement; the opposite of a subjective measurement; measurements cannot be totally objective, because the term "objective" relates to the reliability of measurements, especially the intertester reliability; objectivity and reliability are measured along a continuum. *

Some of the confusion relating to the terms "subjective" and "objective" is due to the manner in which the terms are customarily used. Often in note writing the word **"subjective"** is used to characterize what the patient says, whereas the word **"objective"** is used to characterize what the therapist says. Even though this practice may be widespread and perpetuated through SOAP (subjective, objective, assessment, plan) notes, it represents an inappropriate use of terms. Despite a rather robust body of knowledge dealing with the appropriate uses of the terms "subjective" and "objective," the SOAP approach implies that all the therapist's measurements, because they are listed under "objective," are reliable. We know this is not the case.

The misuse of terms is taken to similar extremes in manual therapy, where the term "objective" is used to describe the physical examination and its results, regardless of how reliable measurements may be. Are assessments of intersegmental mobility objective? Are tests of sacroiliac function objective? In the former case, we do not know the answer, and in the latter case, there are data to suggest we know the answer. Isolated measurements of sacroiliac function do appear to be objective[22]; yet, they are often listed as "objective findings." By using the term "objective" to characterize therapists' statements and examination results, we are actually claiming, usually incorrectly, that our measurements have intertester reliability. The term "objective," when applied to the quality of a measurement, means that a reasonable degree of intertester reliability has been demonstrated.

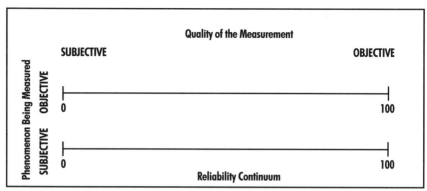

Figure 11. Reliability (Subjective-Objective continuum).

Sometimes the terms "objective" and "subjective" are not used to characterize the quality (ie, reliability) of a measurement, but rather the nature of what is being measured. For example, pain is a subjective phenomenon, but if it is reliably measured, the quality of the measurement is objective. In this case, a subjective phenomenon is measured objectively. Figure 11 shows how the quality of the measurement may be either subjective or objective and how the phenomenon being measured may be either subjective or objective.

Only when the intertester reliability of a measurement is known can the "objectivity" of that measurement be discussed. Too often, assumptions are made about "objectivity" of measurements. We have noted that health care professionals too often assume their measurements are objective, whereas all things reported by patients are subjective. We can also see that when instruments are used to obtain measurements, those measurements are often mistakenly said to be "objective." For example, the use of a dynamometer to measure forces of the quadriceps femoris muscle does not necessarily provide a more objective measurement than does MMT. If, however, we knew that there was greater intertester reliability for the dynamometric measurements than for the MMT grades, then there would be greater objectivity for the dynamometric measurements. In order to make the claim for greater objectivity, data must be provided demonstrating reliability. *Assumptions that a measurement is more likely to be reliable are not a substitute for conducting reliability studies.*

Parallel-Forms Reliability

Sometimes, two or more methods of obtaining a measurement or making a classification develop. We have in physical therapy, for example, at least two methods of obtaining MMT grades.[23,24] In order for the grades obtained with each method to be interpreted and to be used interchangeably, we would need to know whether each method of obtaining a measurement led to the same measurement. The extent to which measurements obtained with different forms of a test agree represents the parallel forms of reliability for those measurements.

Another example of parallel-forms reliability can be found in orthopedic physical therapy. The anterior drawer sign and the pivot shift test (Lachman's test) both are used to assess the structural integrity of the anterior cruciate ligament. If both methods test the same attribute, then the results of both tests should yield the same classification about the ligament. If, however, as proponents of the pivot shift test contend, that test more fully assesses the rotary restraints of the anterior cruciate ligament, then the two tests should not yield the same results. When we believe measurements of the same thing obtained with different methods reflect the same phenomenon, we need to see parallel-forms reliability, but when we contend that one test provides a better or a different kind of measurement, then parallel-forms reliability is not the issue.

In recent years, a variety of dynamometers have been introduced into the marketplace. Do they yield similar measurements? Given the claims of the manufacturers that each has some special characteristics that make it a better machine, one could argue that parallel-forms reliability should not exist. If this is the case, however, any measurement obtained with one device might be fundamentally different than those obtained with a different device. This suggests the potential for chaos in using these measurements and certainly in our ability to find valid uses for these types of measurements. The presence or absence of parallel-forms reliability, therefore, is very relevant for physical therapy practitioners.

Issues Related to Reliability

Among the many factors that can affect the reliability of a measurement is the process of taking a measurement. For example, when a person's muscle is tested on an isokinetic dynamometer, there is a period of time during which the person learns to use the machine. Or, there may be a period during which the person's leg becomes sore because of friction against the machine's lever arm. In either case, the process of taking the measurement will change subsequent measurements. If we cannot correct for these effects, they become sources of error. When the process of taking a measurement affects subsequent measurements, there is **reactivity**. This is defined in the *Standards* as "... *the degree to which the process of taking a test affects a measurement or other measurements taken on the same person in the future.*"* Reactivity can diminish reliability. When administering tests and obtaining measurements, therapists should consider the potential effects of reactivity and attempt to minimize the effects of reactivity.

Judging Reliability

Regardless of the statistical approaches that are used to estimate reliability the issue remains the same: In order to use a measurement, we need to be able to estimate how much of the measurement is error-ridden. We need to know how much of the measurement represents true measurement and how much of it is due to error. If we found that flexion at the glenohumeral joint increased by 45 degrees following treatment, we would certainly feel our treatment was effective. But, how would we feel if we knew there was an average error of 45 degrees in such measurements? We would not be able to determine whether there really was a change. We would not be able to know whether the treatment had any effect. The example illustrates the importance of knowing the estimate of reliability for a measurement. Taking this hypothetical example to further extremes, imagine finding a 95-degree improvement. What would we now think? We could reasonably argue that there was at least a 50-degree improvement, because at best the error could make up only 45 degrees of the measurement. Possibly, there was an even greater treatment effect, but it could be obscured by the error in the measurement.

We need to know the error associated with measurements (ie, the reliability of the measurements) in order to use and interpret those measurements. Sometimes, people will simplify matters by characterizing a measurement as being reliable or not reliable. This is actually a case where transformation of data results in a loss of information. What is happening is that an estimate of error that measures the magnitude of error along an interval or ratio scale is being turned into a categorical statement. As has been noted, any time qualitative measures (interval or ratio) are turned into categorical data, information is lost. This is certainly the case for reliability estimates. When we have an estimate of the error associated with a measurement (as in our shoulder flexion example) we can think about what our measurements mean, we can account for the size of the error—but when we are told that a measurement is, or is not, reliable, we can only just accept or reject the measurement. This latter approach is inappropriate.

By knowing the error associated with a measurement, we can make decisions. For example, you can wonder how much reliability is needed for a measurement, but the answer will depend on how you are using the measurement. In our example, a measurement with a 45-degree error was of little use except in detecting massive changes in ROM (eg, changes greater than 45°). The greater the reliability, the less error, and with less error, a measurement can be used to detect small changes. With large errors, there is less resolution, and the measurement is not useful in examining small changes or characterizing fine details. There is no single acceptable level of reliability. The level depends on how a measurement will be used.

Population-Specific Reliability

We understand the reliability of measurements by examining published research. Test users should pay careful attention to who participated in reliability studies. Two factors that contribute to errors in measurement are the tester and the stability of the phenomenon. In reliability studies, examiners should be similar to those who will use the measurement, and they should measure subjects who are similar to those who will be measured in practice. If one of the world's foremost experts on pulmonary physical therapy could auscultate and classify lung sounds reliably, does that mean anyone else can? Similarly, if it was shown that a group of therapists who were very much like the average clinical therapist could reliably classify lung sounds in patients who were lean, does that mean we could reliably classify lung sounds in persons who were not skinny?

In any reliability study, there are two populations that must be generalized to: the examiners and the persons being examined. In each case, a sample should be drawn that represents the appropriate population. Examining the reliability of measurements of back motion in healthy subjects in order to know the reliability of measurements in patients with low back pain, for example, makes no sense. Reliability estimates that are used by therapists to interpret measurements should have been obtained from patients similar to those being measured. The measurement used to calculate reliability estimates should also have been taken by therapists with similar skill and training as those taking the measurements. The conditions under which the measurements were obtained should also be similar.

In the *Standards*, this issue is dealt with many times. For example, in discussing test manuals, the *Standards* state:

P14.3   *Descriptions of the sample(s) studied in the reliability research must be provided in the test manual.*

   P14.3.1   *Descriptions must be provided in the test manual of how the sample studied in the reliability research was selected.*

   P14.3.2   *The number of subjects studied in the reliability research must be specified in the test manual.*

   P14.3.3   *Descriptions of relevant clinical characteristics of the sample studied in the reliability research must be provided in the test manual. A discussion of how the sample is representative of the population for whom the test is intended should be included in the test manual.*

P14.4   *Descriptions of persons who obtained the measurements in the reliability research (ie, those who were in the role of test users) must be provided in the test manual. Descriptions of their qualifications, competencies, and experiences with the test should be included. Any special information or training given to test users prior to their obtaining the measurements in the study should be described in the test manual.**

The same issue is discussed in the *Standards* relative to the responsibilities of a test user:

U11.   *Test users must be able to describe the population for whom the test was designed. Test users must be able to relate this description to the persons they are testing.**

We have noted the importance of determining whether studies used similar examiners and appropriate patients before we use their estimates of reliability to better understand our measurements. In addition, we have to make sure that we use the same version of the test to obtain measurements before we can claim reliability similar to that reported through research. The *Standards* put it this way:

> **U13.2.** *Test users who deviate from accepted directions for obtaining a measurement should not use published data or documentation relative to reliability and validity to justify their use of the measurement.**

When, however, some alteration must be made, the *Standards* provide guidelines.

> **U45.8.** *Test users who use a variation of a test must indicate, when they report test results, that a variation was used. The test users must note whether they believe that the variation may have affected the quality of their measurements. Test users who believe the variation had a significant effect on the measurement should discuss this belief in all reports of test results.*
>
> **U45.9.** *Test users should report any aspect of the test that may cast doubt on test results (eg, ways in which the person tested differed from the population for which the test was designed or any observation the test user made during testing).**

Issues Relating to Reliability and Validity

Accuracy and Precision

In addition to the terms defined in the *Standards*, other terms are often used to describe measurements. Sometimes these terms add to the confusion. We often talk about the **accuracy** of a measurement or the **precision** of a measurement or a measurement device. The terms "accuracy" and "precision" are often used to characterize how close a measurement comes to a true value, how close it comes to representing the thing being measured. The terms would appear to encompass elements of reliability and validity. Unfortunately, the terms are not easily applied in a consistent fashion to different kinds of measurements.

A good electrocardiogram (ECG) should "accurately" graph the electrical potentials of the heart. Therefore, it would be tempting to say that the ECG was accurate. The purpose of the ECG, however, is to gain insight into whether there is cardiac dysfunction. We know that even in the presence of some normal ECGs, there may be some latent cardiac disease. Although the ECG accurately reflects voltages, it may not accurately reflect the state of health of the heart. When measurements are used to make inferences, the use of the term "accuracy" often becomes problematic because we do not always know whether the word represents the ability of a measurement to reflect some physical phenomenon or to be used to make judgments. The word "precision" also carries the same drawbacks as does the word "accuracy."

These two words, "accuracy" and "precision," are very useful, however, in describing some simple properties of measurement devices. If the ECG did not reflect electrical potentials correctly, it would not have been accurate. When we test whether a dynamometer's measurements reflect applied loads, we are dealing with the accuracy of the device, and to the extent that the device can differentiate small differences in load, we can say the device is precise. If we know that a dynamometer accurately reflects loads, we know something about the mechanical properties of the device. We do not necessarily know what judgments we can make from measurements obtained from patients. The latter is an issue of validity.

Calibration

Some types of test instruments, notably dynamometers, need to be calibrated prior to use. Calibration is the process by which a test instrument is adjusted such that measurements reflect known standards. Adjusting a bathroom scale so that it reads zero when no one is standing on it is a form of calibration. Many instruments need to be calibrated before use. If instruments are not calibrated, measurements will be difficult to interpret, because we will not know what inferences we can make. An uncalibrated instrument will yield values that disagree with those that we should expect, but those measurements can be highly reliable. If that bathroom scale was not on zero but rather was on 10 kg, all subsequent measurements would be 10 kg too high. The consistency of measurements would be unaffected by the failure to calibrate, but the magnitude of the measurements would be affected, as would the validity, unless a correction factor was used.

Technical Aspects of Instruments

Many measurement devices have limited uses. A pain scale written in English should obviously not be used for persons who cannot understand English. Limitations due to more complex and technical aspects of instruments can be equally profound, and test users need to consider how these would affect measurements. Many of the isokinetic devices now being used allow movements in excess of 200°/s. Often therapists want to know the angle at which a given torque occurred. Many of these machines, however, sample the force and angle signals only 100 times per second (100 Hz). Angle-specific measurements at high speeds cannot, therefore, be accurate with this rate of sampling. The Nyquist theorem, which is used to determine how many samples are needed for measurements, suggests that a frequency twice that of what can be expected should be used.[25,26] In other words to have any faith in the angle measurement, we would want a sampling rate of 400 Hz if the movement was 200°/s and a rate of 600 Hz if the movement was at 300°/s.

The dynamometer example highlights the need for test users to understand the technology they use and to understand how it might affect their measurements. This is necessary for both reliability and validity. The *Standards* make the case that test users must understand issues related to technology, but, more importantly, those persons and corporations developing and selling test instruments must describe the technological limitations of their instruments. For example, the *Standards* state that test purveyors (those who sell or promote use of a test) should do the following:

P10. *Test manuals provided by primary purveyors must include descriptions of the test and associated instruments.*

P10.1 *Documentation of relevant technical information regarding performance characteristics of any machines, recording devices, transducers, computer interfaces, and similar instruments must be provided in the test manual.*

P10.2 *Descriptions of how instruments used in the test manipulate or process information in order to obtain the desired measurements must be provided in the test manual.**

Unless test users appreciate the importance of this technical information, it is unlikely that test purveyors will be willing to share this information. Perhaps more importantly, unless test users understand this information, they will not be able to really understand or effectively use the measurements they are obtaining. As the *Standards* note: *"U3.12. Test users must understand the importance of knowing the technical specifications of instruments."**

Summary of Issues Relating to Reliability and Validity

The most important characteristic of a measurement is how valid it is for some purpose. Test users are obligated to consider how they use their measurements and what scientific basis there is for the way they use measurements. In physical therapy, we have begun to develop a body of knowledge about the reliability of many of our measurements. Reliability studies have recently become popular. These studies are important because a measurement that is highly unreliable cannot be very useful. Unfortunately, a measurement can be perfectly reliable, yet absolutely useless. Reliability studies provide some information, but the real necessity is for validity studies.

Researchers are probably concentrating on reliability studies because such studies are easier to conduct than validity studies. If a measurement is highly unreliable, it cannot be valid; therefore, studying the validity of that measurement is not necessary. Properly conducted reliability studies can help us understand the stability of measurements, whether different therapists can obtain similar measurements, and whether different versions of tests can be used interchangeably. Reliability does not tell us whether measurements mean anything, but by knowing the reliability, we can conduct further research and begin to understand our measurements. All test users need to think about both reliability and validity, but ultimately validity is the critical issue.

Statistics Used in the Investigation of Reliability and Validity

Statistics and research designs used to investigate reliability and validity can be quite complex. Recently, for example, the use of generalizability theory[27,28] and item-response theory (Rasch analysis)[29,30] has been gaining popularity for examining the issue of reliability. Any simple discussion of the statistics used in the study of measurement runs the risk of simplifying things to the point of error. The purpose of the following discussion is not to provide a comprehensive view of statistics. That is certainly beyond the scope of a primer. The purpose of this discussion is to illustrate issues associated with the use and interpretation of statistics.

Reliability Indices

In studies of reliability, we often want to determine whether multiple measurements are the same. Similarly, in some investigations of validity, we may want to determine whether measurements obtained from two different tests agree. In each case, we need a statistic that estimates how much two sets of measurements are alike. For quantitative assessments, there are a family of coefficients called **intraclass correlation coefficients (ICCs)** that assess the common variance in sets of measurements.[31-36] The ICC looks at how much variance in sets of measurements is in common; it therefore takes into account levels of disagreement. The ICC takes on a value of 0 to 1. The higher the number, the more the common variance between sets of measurements. There are various forms of the ICC, and the choice of those is beyond the scope of this *Primer*.[31-36]

When we examine reliability, we should care about whether measurements are the same, not whether they are related. The ICC does not directly assess agreement but only common variance, whereas other correlation coefficients look at the relationships (association) among multiple sets of measurements. Reliability is most directly and correctly assessed by looking at agreement. For quantitative measurements, no ideal statistic exists.

There may seem to be no need for a special statistic to assess agreement of quantitative measurements. Intuitively, it would seem that we could calculate how much paired measurements differ and use that calculation as an estimate. For example, if one therapist measured the vital capacity of a patient and another therapist measured the vital capacity, they could determine the percentage difference in their measurements. They could then average those percentage differences to assess agreement across a whole set of vital capacity measurements. An average percentage of agreement would tell them how close their measurements were, but only for the group they measured. Percentage of agreement is a nonprobabilistic (noninferential) statistic that relates only to the sample being measured. Percentage of agreement does not take into account chance agreement, and it does not accurately reflect the level of agreement found in the population.

If two therapists assessed the sitting balance of 20 patients, we could calculate the number of times they agreed and the number of times they disagreed. We might observe, for example, 80% agreement. The problem with using percentage of agreement is that it is a nonprobabilistic (noninferential) estimate of agreement. Percentage of agreement tells you what agreement you obtained for the people you classified; it cannot be used to predict what you could expect when you categorized other persons. For a probabilistic estimate, **Kappa** should be used.

For the assessment of categorical (qualitative) measurements, the most commonly used statistic is some form of Kappa.[37] This statistic is used when we want to determine the extent to which examiners agree when making classifications. When there are few possible choices, however, much of the agreement can occur by chance. Kappa corrects for chance agreement. Imagine we were standing on a New York City street corner and were asked to determine, based on people's accents, whether they were American or some other nationality. Odds are that most of the people we would hear would be Americans. By simply saying "American," we would get relatively good agreement with other assessors, but the agreement would be illusory. The agreement would not represent our ability to classify based on accents, but rather our good fortune to be in a setting where guessing paid off. In the calculation of Kappa, chance agreement is eliminated. Kappa ranges from 0 to 1. The closer Kappa comes to 1, the greater the level of agreement beyond chance.

Sometimes, we make classifications along a continuum. In assessing motion of intervertebral segments, for example, we could judge them to be hypomobile, normal, or hypermobile. In this three-level classification scheme, not all disagreements are equally consequential. If we say hypomobile and someone else examining the same joint says hypermobile, this disagreement is worse than if one said normal and the other said hypomobile. A special version of Kappa, **weighted Kappa**,[38,39] takes into account the consequence of disagreements between examiners. Weighted Kappa is not necessarily used when there are multiple judgments (classifications), but rather when all disagreements are not equally consequential.

Indices of Association

Validity studies often require one measurement to be compared with another measurement. These measurements are frequently in different units. For example, if we were comparing measurements from a new test of ADL with those from an existing test of ADL, we would expect some systematic relationship between scores. One test might have 100 items, the other 200. Agreement in scores, therefore, would not be the issue, but rather some predictable **association** would be expected. The statistic most commonly used to assess association between sets of quantitative measurements is the **Pearson Product-Moment Correlation Coefficient (r)**. The Pearson correlation coefficient can have any value between -1 and +1. A negative value indicates an inverse relationship (as one set of measurements increases, the other decreases), whereas a positive value indicates a direct relationship. A value of

Measurements of Ulcers (mm)

PATIENT NO.	SET 1		SET 2		SET 3	
	1	2	1	2	1	2
1	45	50	45	60.75	45	45
2	55	60	55	74.25	55	55
3	70	75	70	94.50	70	70
4	34	39	34	45.90	34	34
5	56	61	56	75.60	56	56
6	23	28	23	31.05	23	23
7	78	83	78	105.30	78	78
8	89	94	89	120.15	89	89
9	34	39	34	45.90	34	34
10	89	94	89	120.15	89	89

Table 5. Hypothetical Data Illustrating Pearson Product-Moment Correlation Coefficients for Three Sets of Repeated Measurements of Length of Ulcers (in Millimeters)

zero indicates that a set of paired measurements is not systematically related. The Pearson correlation coefficient can be squared to yield another statistic called the **coefficient of determination ($r2$)**. The coefficient of determination estimates the common variance that can be accounted for in two sets of data. Table 5 illustrates some characteristics of the Pearson correlation coefficient.

If we calculated a Pearson correlation coefficient to assess the degree of association between the two measurements in set 1, we would have obtained an $r=1$. Each second measurement increased by 5. This increase represents systematic change. If we calculated a Pearson correlation coefficient to assess the degree of association between the two measurements in set 2, we would have obtained an $r=1$. Each second measurement increased by 35%. This change also represents systematic change. The last set also would give us an $r=1$, but here the two sets of numbers are identical. The Pearson correlation coefficient shows how closely the two sets vary together. In this way, it reflects how strong an association exists between measurements. But this correlation does not tell us anything about the *nature of the relationship*.

If a Pearson correlation coefficient is being used to estimate reliability, we would have no way of knowing how to interpret our measurements. Would a second measurement be expected to normally increase by 5 or by 35%, as we see in the examples? Only when a Pearson correlation coefficient is accompanied by a linear regression equation can we see the **nature of the association** between paired sets of measurements. The **slope** in a linear regression equation estimates the extent of change due to a multiplicative factor, whereas the **intercept** indicates an additive change. A slope of 1 and an intercept of 0 indicate agreement. For our examples, the slopes and intercepts are

For set 1: $r=1$, slope=1, intercept=5.
For set 2: $r=1$, slope=1.35, intercept=0.
For set 3: $r=1$, slope=1, intercept=0.

A second example further illustrates the concepts. A reliability report indicates that when the same person measures limb volume, we could expect perfect agreement ($r=1$), but we would still not know how to interpret any repeated measurements by the same therapist. We would know there was some perfect relationship, but we would not know the nature of that relationship (ie, the arithmetic relationship between first and second measurements). If, however, we knew the slope was 1.2 and the intercept was 0.30, we would expect any second measurement to increase by 20% and by 0.3 units just because we were taking a second measurement. We would know that this change did not reflect a true change in the variable, but rather one we expected as a function of the measurement process. We could then properly interpret our limb volume measurements, because we adjust the measurements by eliminating the systematic error.

The Pearson Product-Moment Correlation Coefficient alone is inadequate for the assessment of reliability of quantitative variables. Similarly, a **Spearman rho**, a correlation for ordinal data, does not address the issue of whether ordinal classifications agree. The Spearman rho assesses the extent to which two sets of ranked data relate to each other. Spearman rho is very useful for looking at relationships between sets of ordinal data, as we often need to do in validity studies, but when we need to assess agreement of such data, Kappa more clearly addresses the issue.

Indices of Measurement Error

Among measurement experts, there is little disagreement that the ideal statistic for estimating the error associated with reliability is the **standard error of the measurement (SEM).**[16] This statistic is expressed in units of the measurement and, therefore, can be easily used in most settings. We know that 95% of all scores will lie between ± 2 SEMs. This is because the SEM, which is based on the standard deviation, has properties similiar to those of the standard deviation. If we knew that the torque a person could generate on a low back testing machine was 400 Nm and that the SEM was 23 Nm, we would know that we had a 95% chance of being correct when we assumed that the person's true measurement was somewhere between 354 Nm and 446 Nm (400-[2x23]) to (400+([2x23]).

Although the SEM is a useful statistic and is commonly used in many fields to estimate reliability (particularly in psychology), there has been little use of this statistic in physical therapy. The SEM is a relatively conservative probabilistic statistic, and in order to estimate reliability, large samples are needed when using the SEM. When small samples are studied, the SEM tends to greatly overestimate the error. Davis[40] argues that for calculations of SEM, at least 400 measurements should be used. Nunnally[41] illustrates measurement error by using examples with 300 measurements. Until larger samples are used in physical therapy research in reliability, the SEM will remain a desired, but impractical, statistic. In view of the usefulness and theoretical soundness of the SEM, we can only hope that in the future researchers will use sufficiently large samples to allow for the use of the SEM.

Sometimes, in an effort to estimate error, the **coefficient of variation (CV)** is reported. The CV is the standard deviation expressed as a percentage of the mean (CV=[SD/mean]x100). Can this statistic reflect reliability? Not really. If we measure a group of subjects, each measurement will consist of a true component and some error. Therefore, the standard deviation will reflect the variability of measurements among subjects and, to some extent, error in measurements. The standard deviation and the related CV reflect variability of measurements within a sample, not measurement error. If, however, no variability was expected in the measurement, as would occur with 100 repeated measurements of the area of a tabletop, then all variability would represent error. Under these special circumstance, the CV could be used to estimate error, but it would be a nonprobabilistic (noninferential) estimate. When used to estimate reliability, the CV describes the variability of a sample.

Terms Used to Describe Reliability and Validity Estimates

Sometimes research on reliability or validity will refer to an index of reliability, a coefficient of reliability, or an index of validity. Many statistics can be used to examine the issues of reliability and validity. There is no one statistical method. Authors who write of reliability coefficients or validity coefficients are describing how they used a statistic and not what statistic was used. This type of terminology should be used with caution, because estimates of reliability or validity can be interpreted only if we know what statistic was used to generate the estimate.

References

1　McKenzie RA. *The Lumbar Spine: Mechanical Diagnosis and Therapy.* Waikanae, New Zealand: Spinal Publications Ltd; 1981.

2　*American Heritage Dictionary.* Boston, Mass: Houghton Mifflin Co; 1986.

3　Wynn-Parry CB. Various movements (trick movements). In: Licht S, ed. *Therapeutic Exercise.* 2nd ed. Baltimore, Md: Williams & Wilkins; 1965:117-127.

4　Delitto A. Subjective measures and clinical decision making. *Phys Ther.* 1989;69:585-589.

5　Fairbanks JCT, Couper J, Davies JB, et al. The Oswestry Low Back Pain Disability Questionnaire. *Physiotherapy.* 1980;66:271-273.

6　Mahoney FT, Barthel DW. Functional evaluation: the Barthel Index. *Md Med J.* 1965;14:61-65.

7　Chandler LS, Andrews MS, Swanson MW. *The Movement Assessment of Infants: A Manual.* Rolling Bay, Wash: Chandler, Andrews & Swanson; 1980.

8　Harris SR, Haley SM, Tada WL, Swanson MW. Reliability of observational measures of the Movement Assessment of Infants. *Phys Ther.* 1984;64:471-475.

9　Cohen J, Cohen P. *Applied Multiple Regression: Correlation Analysis for the Behavioral Sciences.* 2nd ed. Hillsdale, NJ: Lawrence Erlbaum Associates Inc; 1983:72-73, 413-423.

10　Safrit MJ, Wood TM. *Measurement Concepts in Physical Education and Exercise Science.* Champaign, Ill: Human Kinetics Publishers Inc; 1989: chap 10.

11　Cronbach LJ, Furby L. How should we measure "change"—or should we? *Psychol Bull.* 1970;74: 68-80.

12　Linn RL, Slinde JA. The determination of significance of change between pre- and post-testing periods. *Review of Educational Research.* 1977;47:121-150.

13　Snedecor GW, Cochran WG. *Statistical Methods.* 6th ed. Ames, Iowa: Iowa University Press; 1967: chap 3.

14　Besag FP, Besag PL. *Statistics for the Helping Professions.* Beverly Hills, Calif: Sage Publications; 1985.

15　Gerhardt JJ, Russe OA. *International SFTR Method of Measuring and Recording Joint Motion.* Bern, Switzerland: Hans Huber AG; 1975.

16　Anastasi A. *Psychological Testing.* 6th ed. New York, NY: Macmillan Publishing Co; 1988:92-94.

17　Kerlinger FN. *Foundations of Behavioral Research.* 2nd ed. New York, NY: Holt, Rinehart and Winston, Inc; 1986: chap 8.

18　Lovett RW. *The Treatment of Infantile Paralysis.* 2nd ed. Philadelphia, Pa: P Blakiston & Son Co; 1917.

19　Helms CA. *Fundamentals of Skeletal Radiology.* Philadelphia, Pa: WB Saunders Co; 1989.

20　Sinacore DR, Ehsani AA. Measurements in cardiovascular function. In: Rothstein JM, ed. *Measurement in Physical Therapy.* New York, NY: Churchill Livingstone Inc; 1985:255-280.

21　Rothstein JM, Roy SH, Wolf SL. *Rehabilitation Specialist's Handbook.* Philadelphia, Pa: FA Davis Co; 1991:67-68.

22　Potter N, Rothstein JM. Intertester reliability for selected clinical tests of the sacroiliac joint. *Phys Ther.* 1985;65:1671-1675.

23　Kendall FP, McCreary EK, Provance PG. *Muscles: Testing and Function.* 4th ed. Baltimore, Md: Williams & Wilkins; 1993.

24　Daniels L, Worthingham C. *Muscle Testing: Techniques of Manual Examination.* 5th ed. Philadelphia, Pa: WB Saunders Co; 1986.

25 Winter DA. *Biomechanics of Human Movement*. New York, NY: John Wiley & Sons Inc; 1979:9-46.

26 Nyquist H. Regeneration theory. Reprinted in: MacFarlance AGJ, ed. *Frequency Response Methods in Control Systems*. New York, NY: IEEE Press; 1979.

27 Campbell JP. Psychometric theory. In: Dunnette MD, ed. *Handbook of Industrial and Organizational Psychology*. Chicago, Ill: Rand McNally & Co; 1976.

28 Mitchell SK. Interobserver agreement: reliability and generalizability of data collected in observational studies. *Psychol Bull*. 1979;86:376-390.

29 Rasch G. *Probabilistic Models for Some Intelligence and Attainment Tests*. Chicago, Ill: University of Chicago Press; 1980.

30 Wright BD, Stone MH. *Best Test Design: Rasch Measurement*. Chicago, Ill: MESA Press; 1979.

31 Shrout PE, Fleiss JL. Intraclass correlations: uses in assessing rater reliability. *Psychol Bull*. 1979;86:421-428.

32 Bartko JJ. The intraclass correlation coefficient as a measure of reliability. *Psychol Rep*. 1966;19:3-11.

33 Bartko JJ, Carpenter WT. On the methods of theory of reliability. *J Nerv Ment Dis*. 1976;163:307-317.

34 Bartko JJ. On various intraclass correlations. *Psychol Bull*. 1976;83:762-765.

35 Lahey MA, Downey RG, Saal FE. Intraclass correlations: there is more there than meets the eye. *Psychol Bull*. 1983;93:586-595.

36 Krebs DE. Intraclass correlation coefficients: use and calculation. *Phys Ther*. 1984;64:1581-1584.

37 Cohen J. Coefficient of agreement for nominal scales. *Educational and Psychological Measurement*. 1960;20:37-46.

38 Cohen J. Weighted Kappa: nominal scale agreement with provision for scaled disagreement or partial credit. *Psychol Bull*. 1968;70:213-220.

39 Fleiss JL, Cohen J, Everett BS. Large sample standard errors of Kappa and weighted Kappa. *Psychol Bull*. 1969;72:323-327.

40 Davis FB. *Educational Measurements and Their Interpretation*. Belmont, Calif: Wadsworth Publishing Co Inc; 1964:339.

41 Nunnally JC. *Psychometric Theory*. New York, NY: McGraw-Hill Book Co; 1967:172-210.

Index to Tables and Figures

Appendix

Standards for Tests and Measurements in Physical Therapy Practice

Standards for Tests and Measurements in Physical Therapy Practice

(Reprinted from *Physical Therapy*, August 1991, Volume 71, Number 8, pages 589-621)[†]

Table of Contents

† *Reprinted with permission of the American Physical Therapy Association.*

Preface

The Standards for Tests and Measurements in Physical Therapy Practice is a cohesive and well-organized document, complete with operational definitions and primer. During a first reading, one might readily conclude that the entire work is an academic treatise, esoteric in nature and dedicated to a select handful of clinicians with the intellectual capacity and interest to glean meaning from its organization. These Standards, however, represent far more than can be processed by a cursory glance or a preoccupied mind.

As defined by the Board of Directors of the American Physical Therapy Association (November 1984), a standard is an approved, binding, general statement of requirement used to judge quality of action or activity. As such, standards are accessible to the lay and health professional public for their scrutiny and criticism. To mature from concept to finality, therefore, implies a honing process of utmost delicateness and comprehension, for to expose our standards of measurements and tests to those who may judge us is to reveal an identity perhaps unknown to or misunderstood by such parties. At a time in which physical therapists seek greater autonomy in clinical decision making, standards indeed do become the palettes from which our destiny is stroked.

With this perspective in mind, a task force of the Committee on Research was created in 1987 to develop standards for tests and measures used commonly in physical therapy practice. This task force, coordinated by Jules Rothstein, included Suzann Campbell, John Echternach, Alan Jette, Harry Knecht, and the late Steven Rose. The group sought to produce standards that addressed logical requirements for measurement, reproduction of test results, and interpretation and use of such results. All materials were reviewed by representatives of Sections and Specialty Councils; physical therapists primarily in education, research, or practice environments; and external experts. Collectively, these professionals recognized that we are at risk in any working environment unless our tests and measurements are creditable and specifically identifiable with our clinical activities. Standards were needed to improve the quality of our practice, lend a unifying perspective to the instruction of measurements to our students, and enhance the rigor of our research activities. The standards necessary to meet these requirements had to be unique to physical therapy and easily associated with our professional skills by practitioners, faculty, and students; medical groups who have vested interests in the quality of physical rehabilitation services; and third-party payers who assess the rigor of our interventions and the meaning of our quantitative values.

After 4 years and untold hours of labor, these Standards are a reality. They promote consistency and imply unification of purpose. These traits are needed at a time when many might forsake the quality inherent in consistency of measurement for the speed and sloppiness so often ensconced in uncontrolled profit rampages. What are our options? One can choose to ignore the Standards for Tests and Measurements in Physical Therapy Practice, not out of disrespect or even ignorance, but out of indifference. The consequences are patently clear. Our failure to implement these Standards could diminish the singularity of our identity—not only among ourselves and our medical colleagues, but also, more relevantly, among those who must render decisions about our services and livelihood. On the other hand, a conscientious effort to comprehend, digest, and implement our adopted Standards is a true precursor in our quest to stand alone as a unique and esoteric profession. So seek wisdom and guidance from these Standards, recognizing that their intent is neither total compliance nor comprehension at a first reading, but absorption and integration into practice upon multiple readings. In the final analysis, those medical services that will stand the test of time will be characterized by comprehensible quantification performed with uncompromising quality.

Steven L Wolf, PhD, PT, FAPTA
Chairman, Advisory Council on Research to the Board of Directors, APTA

The need for and value of standards for tests and measurements is clear—physical therapists must have a more scientific basis for practice. We test and measure in our daily practice, yet the validity and reliability of some of these tests may be questioned. With this document, we have guidelines to determine the quality of our tests and measurements.

Measurements are fundamental to the practice of physical therapy. We need to sit back and look at what we do each day, and strive for the quality we are capable of providing. Meaningful and useful measurements are important if we, as physical therapists, are to be recognized as credible health care providers.

Achieving a high quality of physical therapy practice requires us to evaluate the client, selecting and administering a variety of tests and measurements. We take our findings, interpret the data, and establish a baseline for the client's status. We then develop plans for therapeutic intervention that will achieve the goals we have set for the client. But how objective and accurate are those findings? How reliable? How valid? Can we select the appropriate interventions if our assessments are in question?

Standards provide the foundation for assessment of the quality of our practice. We use a variety of quality assurance methodologies to determine the degree to which the standards are met, and we take actions to improve the care when standards are not met. Quality assurance is the responsibility of every physical therapist, as well as the responsibility of the profession as a whole. Quality assurance continues to be an evolving process. The tools may change, but the objective remains the same: to improve patient care.

The physical therapy evaluation is the foundation for the measurement of the outcome of our therapeutic intervention. And we must measure these outcomes. In the past, quality assurance activities have focused more on the structure and process of our services. With the spiraling cost of health care in the United States, we must demonstrate the effectiveness and efficiency of our treatment. Quality assurance studies with an outcome focus can provide a measure of our progress toward achieving that goal.

We have our Standards of Practice adopted by the House of Delegates of the American Physical Therapy Association, and these standards assist us in our quality assurance mechanisms. Now, we have the Standards for Tests and Measurements in Physical Therapy Practice to assist us in ensuring the quality of our physical therapy evaluation. Clinicians must take these criteria and try to incorporate them into their daily practice.

The Task Force on Standards for Measurement in Physical Therapy has completed a complex task in advancing our knowledge and has provided a cornerstone of objective, reliable, and standardized tests and measurements. The Task Force members are to be commended for their hard work.

Elizabeth Gaynor, MS, PT
Chairperson, Committee on Physical Therapy Practice

Dedication

The members of the American Physical Therapy Association's Task Force on Measurement dedicate this document to Dr Steven J Rose, who died before the document was completed. Dr Rose was a visionary within physical therapy. He saw the need for standards for tests and measurements and welcomed the creation of a task force. He gladly accepted a position on the task force, despite the fact that he was ill. During the early phases of writing this document, he displayed remarkable courage, overcoming pain and disability to attend meetings. He was a vigorous participant in discussions. We note with pride his remarks that his excitement about this project led him to work longer and harder than he thought he could and that, in the midst of task force business, he even forgot about his pain and fatigue. Dr Rose's brilliant mind, his penchant for playing the devil's advocate, and his commitment to excellence were missed in the latter stages of this project. His spirit, however, remains in his many contributions to the Standards and accompanying documents and in the way these documents attempt to combine science and practice, Dr Rose's two great loves.

Introduction

Examination of physical therapy practice demonstrates the growing importance of measurement. Walking through a physical therapy clinic, you may observe a patient's range of motion being measured, or you may see a therapist testing the inspiratory capacity of a patient. Other therapists may be measuring the developmental status of a child or the accessory motion of the knee joint in a postsurgical patient. Still other therapists may be measuring the functional status of a patient with hemiplegia. Physical therapists need to obtain measurements because they make decisions, offer consultative opinions, and document changes in patient status.

This document, Standards for Tests and Measurements in Physical Therapy Practice, has been prepared because of the growing importance of measurement in physical therapy. Measurements are taken to provide information, but the result may be misinformation if the quality of measurements is not ensured. The purpose of this document is to provide standards that will help ensure the quality of measurements. These Standards are tools for practitioners. They are designed to provide guidelines that practitioners can use when they take measurements. The Standards are meant to represent the best in measurement and are not intended to hinder practice by establishing rigid rules that interfere with patient care. The Standards also demonstrate to society the commitment of physical therapists to practice in a credible and scientific manner. The Standards reflect our profession's humanistic commitment to provide the highest quality of care to our patients. The Standards include a section on research. The Standards, however, are primarily related to practice. They set how measurements should be used in clinical practice. Through the use of the Standards, therapists can, in their practice settings, deliver more effective care and document the results of treatment.

As clinicians, we cannot practice unless we take measurements. We need measurements in order to classify and describe patients, plan treatments, predict outcomes, document the results of treatments, and determine when to refer patients to other practitioners. We may wonder how much more effectively we might practice if we knew more about our measurements, for example, if we knew when we should rely on our measurements and when we should seek confirming information. In addition to needing measurements for decision making, we need measurements in order to document what we are doing. In the face of shrinking resources for health care, society is no longer willing to accept on good faith alone the benefit of what we physical therapists do for our patients. Even widely accepted treatments may, in the future, become suspect if the measurements that justify these treatments are shown to be questionable.

This is an age when documentation, efficacy, and cost-effectiveness are increasingly important to those who control the reimbursement for all of health care, including physical therapy. Measurement will play an increasing role in determining who gets paid for doing what to whom, and for how long. Documentation with measurements of high quality may be the only way we physical therapists can ensure that our services will be available to persons who need these services. Physical therapy as a form of health care is at risk unless the results of physical therapy are judged to be worthwhile, not only by physical therapists and consumers of physical therapy, but also by third-party payers and corporate-world purchasers of health care. Some or much of what is being done in physical therapy could be denied reimbursement if we do not satisfactorily document the efficacy and cost-effectiveness of treatment. Without such reimbursement, physical therapy services could be denied to the very people who need our services the most. Proper attention to the quality of measurement in clinical practice will, therefore, not only ensure our profession's continued growth but also protect our patients.

Growth in the profession of physical therapy has taken place even though our profession has had no accepted standards for measurement and despite the fact that few education programs have prepared new therapists to understand what constitutes good measurement.

Continued growth cannot be ensured unless the state of our measurements changes—and unless it changes soon. In March of 1986, the Board of Directors of the American Physical Therapy Association (APTA) recognized the need to improve the state of measurement in physical therapy. The Board made improved measurement a major goal of the Association.

Because resources in clinical measurement were limited, the Board called upon the Research Committee to develop a proposal for the development of Standards for Measurement in Physical Therapy. In August of 1987, the Research Committee, after consulting with experts on clinical measurement, developed a proposal for the development of Standards for Measurement in Physical Therapy. In November of 1987, the Board funded the proposal and made a commitment to a 2-year effort that would culminate in the publication of these Standards. The Task Force on Standards for Measurement in Physical Therapy was appointed to carry out this mission.

Physical therapy is not the first profession to recognize the need to improve the quality of its measurements. The American Psychological Association (APA) has been publishing monographs on standards in testing since 1954. The American Educational Research Association and the National Council on Measurement in Education joined forces with the APA in the mid-1960s and formed a joint committee that wrote Standards for Educational and Psychological Tests and Manuals. A 1966 version of the Standards has been revised twice, with the most recent edition published in 1985.

One of the first acts of the Task Force members was to examine the APA manual. The APA Standards are a primary source of information on measurement. The members of the Task Force agreed, however, that while the APA document contained a great deal of useful information, it was not directly applicable to physical therapy. Many of the measurement problems in physical therapy are unique. Physical therapists use measurements that are based on the behavioral, biological, and physical sciences. The scope of measurements in physical therapy is extraordinary. Questionnaires are used by therapists, as are manual muscle testing, developmental testing, postural evaluations, instrumented muscle testing, movement analysis, and a whole variety of other tests. Instruments vary from paper and pencil, to the therapist's hands, to complex computer-based machines with elaborate peripheral devices. We concluded that clinicians needed standards written by physical therapists for physical therapy practitioners. The Task Force, therefore, set out to develop Standards specifically for physical therapy. In developing these Standards, the Task Force was aware that most physical therapists receive little or no training in the science of measurement. The Task Force agreed that the final document must be sufficiently comprehensive to cover the vast expanse of physical therapy measurements and that it must also be practical.

The process of developing standards began with the entire Task Force considering philosophical and practical issues during 2 days of often heated, and always thorough, discussion. After the Task Force worked out basic concepts, the writing of the Standards was delegated to a three-member Working Group (Jules M Rothstein, Task Force coordinator; John L Echternach; and Harry G Knecht). The Working Group developed a draft document that was initially reviewed by the rest of the Task Force. The draft was revised. The present version has been revised on feedback from the physical therapy community, as well as on feedback from other interested parties and from experts on measurement.

In the training of physical therapists, measurement has all too often been equated with research. Concerns about the quality of measurements are, at times mistakenly, thought to relate to research and not to practice. Because therapists need help with the basic science of measurement, a primer on measurement has been prepared to complement the Standards. The purposes of the primer are to provide physical therapists with explanations of basic concepts and to explore issues related to measurement. Eugene Michels, who began work with the Task Force as an APTA staff member, wrote the initial draft of the primer. The primer is a tool that can be used to help understand not only the Standards, but also issues related to tests and measurements themselves. The primer is an independent, but complementary, document of the Standards.

The Standards include a glossary. The glossary defines terms as they are used in the Standards. The glossary allows readers to see how these terms were used by the authors of the Standards. The Task Force made every effort to avoid creating new terms and to avoid using jargon. The glossary is meant solely as a source for materials in the Standards; it is not a general measurement glossary. Whenever possible, the terms used and defined are those commonly found in the measurement literature. Clinicians may find many of the terms unfamiliar at first, but the Task Force believes that, through use of the glossary and the primer, the Standards can be understood and used by all therapists. The Task Force also recognizes that many physical therapists will have to make a commitment of time and effort to learn these new terms and to learn about measurement. In the future, these terms will be more commonplace in the clinical literature of physical therapy.

The Standards are meant to foster the continued growth of high-quality care in physical therapy. They are highly specific in describing what should be done to ensure meaningful and useful measurements. Part of the Standards provides long-overdue guidance to persons developing tests and to persons teaching about testing. No longer will clinicians independently have to ask purveyors of tests to supply vital information. The Standards specify what the providers should provide.

The Standards consist of five sections. The first three sections specify what is expected of test purveyors. Three categories of purveyors are described: primary purveyors, who originate tests; secondary purveyors, who conduct research and advocate the use of tests; and tertiary purveyors, who are teachers. The fourth section contains the Standards for Test Users—physical therapists. The fifth section describes standards for ensuring integrity in measurement studies. This last section is adapted from the APTA's Standards for Integrity in Physical Therapy Research.

The Task Force originally had hoped to generate a series of guidelines that would be few in number and "user friendly." Early versions of the Standards proved that this was impossible. Attempts to generate fewer sections and a more multipurpose document resulted in a cumbersome set of standards that was difficult to apply. Because this is the first document of its type in physical therapy and because of the nature of the subject, we found that the Standards needed to be comprehensive and to contain detailed specifications. We found that when we attempted to produce briefer versions of the Standards and when we attempted to use fewer measurement terms, our drafts were unclear and could not be used as references. The Standards, although they are advisory, may read like a rule book. Such books are not easily read, nor are they commonly read from cover to cover. We chose to separate the Standards into sections, each for a specific audience. For example, physical therapists will usually be acting as test users and should read and consult the section designed for them. Therapists may, however, on occasion want to know what they should expect from purveyors of tests. When this need is recognized, they can consult the appropriate purveyor section.

In the Standards, the word "must" appears frequently. The Task Force consciously adopted the use of this word to provide a clear message about measurement. This message is that physical therapists who make decisions about measurements and their uses should understand that the use of the best measurements possible is obligatory. It is equally important to understand other ideas in this context. There is no intention to have anyone act as an enforcer of the Standards. The Standards represent an ideal; they represent a guide that therapists can use in their professional conduct. Measurements in physical therapy will improve when each therapist considers his or her own responsibility regarding the Standards.

The Standards provide a framework for professional decisions. They are optimal guidelines, not fixed, inviolate rules. Because standards are by their very nature statements of optimal characteristics, there is still considerable room for judgment.* Task Force members believe that measurements that fail to meet the Standards are less than ideal and that every effort should be made to avoid using such measurements. When that is not possible, clinical practice cannot wait and testing will usually have to proceed; however, physical therapists should be aware of and should acknowledge the limitations of the measurements they are using. The Standards should also heighten an awareness that the business of measurement should not be taken casually. The development of tests and measurements takes commitment and is often an arduous process that is marked by periods of testing and refinement. Therefore, although tests cannot necessarily meet all of the Standards, it is the responsibility of all persons promoting and using tests and measurements to make sure that reasonably acceptable adherence to the Standards occurs and that future efforts will be made at refinement.

This document is open to review. The published Standards for Tests and Measurements in Physical Therapy Practice represent only the beginning of an important effort. As the Standards continue to evolve, we hope that physical therapists will aid that endeavor by sharing with us their impressions and experiences with the Standards.

We believe that the Standards will become an essential part of physical therapy practice. Knowledge of measurement is no less important for clinical practice than is knowledge of anatomy, kinesiology, physiology, or psychology. All of these areas, including measurement, provide the scientific foundation for effective clinical practice. These are the profession's Standards, and, as such, they are a means of ensuring better care for our patients and of ensuring that physical therapists play an important role in the delivery of health care services.

*The Standards are not intended to codify, explain, modify, or replace any part of the ethical principles in the APTA's Code of Ethics or any of the interpretations in the Guide for Professional Conduct, which is issued by the Association's Judicial Committee.

Glossary of Terms Used in the Standards

The glossary describes terms as they are used in the Standards. The glossary is not meant to be all-inclusive, but rather to provide definitions for the terms as they are used in the Standards. For further information about the terms, related concepts, or other terms used in measurement, consult the Primer.

Alternate-forms (parallel-forms) reliability: see **reliability**

Assessment: measurement, quantification, or placing a value or label on something; assessment is often confused with evaluation; an assessment results from the act of assessing (see **evaluation** and **examination**)

Attribute: a variable; a characteristic or quality that is measured

Classification (categorization): assignment of an individual or an entity to a group; assignment is based on rules; groups are defined so that they allow all pertinent entities or individuals to belong to the defined groups (classes or categories are exhaustive) and so that they allow entities or individuals to belong to only one possible group (classes or categories are mutually exclusive)

Clinical decision: a determination that relates to direct patient care, indirect patient care, acceptance of patients for treatment, and whether patients should be referred to other practitioners (this definition is modified from that presented by Charles Magistro at a conference on Clinical Decision Making held under APTA auspices in October 1988 in Lake of the Ozarks, Missouri); a diagnosis that leads to therapist to take an action is a form of a clinical decision; clinical decisions result in actions; when direct supporting evidence for clinical decisions is lacking, such decisions are based on clinical opinions

Clinical opinion: a belief or idea that a physical therapist holds regarding a patient; this opinion may be based on the use of tests and measurements, but is not directly supported by evidence relating to those tests and measurements; clinical opinions are based on the therapist's evaluation of available information; clinical decisions (ie, determinations that cause the therapist to take an action) that are based on the therapist's synthesis of information are based on the clinical opinions of that therapist

Concurrent validity; see **validity**

Construct: a concept developed for the purpose of measurement; support for the construct is through logical argumentation based on the theoretical and research evidence (see construct validity listed under validity)

Construct validity: see **validity**

Content validity: see **validity**

Criterion-based (criterion-related) validity: see **validity**

Data: synonymous with measurements (see **measurement**)

Derived measurement: a measurement of an attribute that is obtained as the result of a mathematical operation applied to an existing measurement of some other attribute; an example is the measurement of leg-length difference, which is derived by subtracting one leg-length measurement from another

Evaluation: a judgment based on a measurement; often confused with assessment and examination (see **assessment** and **examination**); evaluations are judgments of the value or worth of something

Examination: a test or a group of tests used for the purpose of obtaining measurements or data (see **assessment** and **evaluation**)

False negatives: persons who test negatively for some attribute but who, in fact, have that attribute (see **true negatives**)

False positives: persons who test positively for some attribute but who, in fact, do not have that attribute (see **true positives**)

Instrument: a machine, a questionnaire, or any device that is used as part of, or as a test to obtain, measurements

Internal consistency: see **reliability**

Intertester reliability: see **reliability**

Intratester reliability: see **reliability**

Measure: the act of obtaining a measurement (datum)

Measurement: the numeral assigned to an object, event, or person or the class (category) to which an object, event, or person is assigned according to rules

Normalization: a process that yields a new or transformed measurement that is mathematically derived to change the distribution of measurements; normalization procedures are often used to change the distribution of data to make the distribution more congruent with a bell-shaped (or normal) curve

Objective measurement: a measurement that is not affected by some aspect of the person obtaining the measurement; the opposite of a subjective measurement (see **subjective measurement**); measurements cannot be totally objective, because the term "objective" relates to the reliability of measurements, especially in the intertester reliability; objectivity and reliability are measured along a continuum

Operational definition: a set of procedures that guides the process of obtaining a measurement; includes descriptions of the attribute that is to be measured, the conditions under which the measurement is to be taken, and the actions that are to be taken in order to obtain the measurement

Parallel-forms (alternate-forms) reliability: see **reliability**

Practicality of a test: the usefulness of a test based on issues relating to personnel, time, equipment, cost of administration, and impact on the person taking a test

Predictive validity: see **validity**

Predictive value of a measurement: the degree of certainty that can be associated with a positive or negative finding (measurement) obtained on a diagnostic test; the predictive value of a positive measurement is the ratio formed by dividing the number of true positives by the number of all positive findings; the predictive value of a negative measurement is the ratio formed by dividing the number of true negatives by the number of all negative findings

Prescriptive validity: see **validity**

Primary purveyor: see **purveyor**

Purveyor: any person (or organization) who develops a test or any person (or organization) who offers, promotes, or requires the use of a test; a purveyor is also a person who advocates use of specific tests through the publication of research or scholarly articles or through teaching

> *Primary purveyor:* a person who develops, promotes, or requires that use of tests; this definition includes persons within clinical institutions who require the use of specific tests; persons who conduct continuing education courses in which a major component involves the advocacy of the use of specific testing procedures are primary purveyors; any person (or organization) who promotes (advocates) the use of tests by selling testing equipment, manuals, books, or similar materials is a primary purveyor; in the case of books or articles that serve as test manuals, the primary purveyor is the author; persons who sell instruments that may be used for testing, but who do not describe or advocate specific testing procedures, are not purveyors (see **purveyor**, *secondary purveyor*, and *tertiary purveyor*)

> *Secondary purveyor:* any researcher or other person who publishes a scholarly work that examines aspects of tests and who, in that scholarly work, suggests (advocates) that a test be used; a secondary purveyor is not the initial source of information on a test (ie, did not supply the manual or the original information on the test) (see **purveyor**, *primary purveyor*, and *tertiary purveyor*)

> *Tertiary purveyor:* any person who teaches or prepares instructional material that describes specific tests or specific uses of measurements; this definition includes, but is not limited to, persons teaching in academic institutions, clinical educators, and continuing educators who are not acting in the role of primary or secondary purveyors (see **purveyor**, *primary purveyor*, and *secondary purveyor*)

Reactivity: the degree to which the process of taking a test affects a measurement or other measurements taken on the same person in the future; examples are learning and physiological effects of taking tests

Reliability: the consistency or repeatability of measurements; the degree to which measurements are error-free and the degree to which repeated measurements will agree

> *Internal consistency:* the extent to which items or elements that contribute to a measurement reflect one basic phenomenon or dimension

> *Intertester reliability:* the consistency or equivalence of measurements when more than one person takes the measurements; indicates agreement of measurements taken by different examiners

> *Intratester reliability:* the consistency or equivalence of measurements when one person takes repeated measurements separated in time; indicates agreement in measurements over time

> *Parallel-forms (alternate-forms) reliability:* the consistency or agreement of measurements obtained with different (alternative) forms of a test; indicates whether measurements obtained with different forms of a test can be used interchangeably

> *Test-retest reliability:* the consistency or repeated measurements separated in time; indicates stability (reliability) over time

Score (grade): the numeric (quantitative) or verbal (qualitative) descriptor used to characterize the result of a test; a score is a measurement (see measurement)

Secondary purveyor: see **purveyor**

Sensitivity of a test: an indication of how well a diagnostic test identifies people who should have a positive finding; the numerical representation of sensitivity is a ratio formed by dividing the number of persons with a true-positive response on a test by the number of persons who should have had a positive response (ie, the number of persons who are known to have properties that would indicate that they should test positive)

Specificity of a test: an indication of how well a diagnostic test identifies people who should have a negative finding; the numerical representation of specificity is a ratio formed by dividing the number of persons with a true-negative response on a test by the number of persons who should have had a negative response (ie, the number of persons who are known to have properties that would indicate that they should test negative)

Standardization: a process by which a score is converted (transformed) into a relative score by using indices of central tendency and variability; a commonly used standardized score is the z score; the term "standardization" is also used to describe the process of systematization of the methods used to obtain a measurement; the process of standardization, however, does not ensure reliability, because reliability can only be determined through the collection of data (see **reliability**)

Subjective measurement: a measurement that is affected by some aspect of the person obtaining the measurement (contrasts with **objective measurement**); subjectivity relates to the reliability of measurements, especially the intertester reliability; the more subjective the measurement, the less reliable the measurement; subjectivity, like reliability, is measured along a continuum

Tertiary purveyor: see **purveyor**

Test: a procedure or set of procedures that is used to obtain measurements (data); the procedures may require the use of instruments

Test manual: a booklet or book prepared by a primary test purveyor to guide the process of obtaining a measurement and to provide documentation and justification for the test

Test setting: the environment in which a test is given, including the physical setting and the characteristics of that setting

Test user: one who chooses tests, interprets test scores, or makes decisions based on test scores (this definition is from *Standards for Educational and Psychological Tests; American Psychological Association,* Washington, DC, 1974, page 1)

Test-retest reliability: see **reliability**

Transformation of measurements: the application of a mathematical operation for the purpose of changing the value or distribution of measurements, such as is done in the process of standardization or normalization

True negatives: persons who test negatively for some attribute and who, in fact, do not have that attribute (see **false negatives**)

True positives: persons who test positively for some attribute and who, in fact, have that attribute (see **false positives**)

Validity: the degree to which a useful (meaningful) interpretation can be inferred from a measurement

Concurrent validity: a form of criterion-based validity in which an inferred interpretation is justified by comparing a measurement with supporting evidence that was obtained at approximately the same time as the measurement being validated

Construct validity: the conceptual (theoretical) basis for using a measurement to make an inferred interpretation; evidence for construct validity is through logical argumentation based on theoretical and research evidence (see **construct**)

Content validity: a form of validity that deals with the extent to which a measurement is judged to reflect the meaningful elements of a construct and not any extraneous elements

Criterion-based (criterion-related) validity: three forms of criterion-based validity exist: concurrent validity, predictive validity, and prescriptive validity; the common element is that, with each of these forms of validity, the correctness of an inferred interpretation can be tested by comparing a measurement with either a different measurement or data obtained by other forms of testing

Predictive validity: a form of criterion-based validity in which an inferred interpretation is justified by comparing a measurement with supporting evidence that is obtained at a later point in time; examines the justification of using a measurement to say something about future events or conditions

Prescriptive validity: a form of criterion-based validity in which the inferred interpretation of a measurement is the determination of the form of treatment a person is to receive; prescriptive validity is justified based on the successful outcome of the chosen treatment

Standards for Tests and Measurements in Physical Therapy Practice

Standards for Primary Test Purveyors (indicated with a P)

The Standards in this section describe requirements for primary purveyors of tests. The following is the definition of a primary purveyor.

Primary purveyor: a person who develops, promotes, or requires the use of tests; this definition includes persons within clinical institutions who require the use of specific tests; persons who conduct continuing education courses in which a major component involves the advocacy of the use of specific testing procedures are primary purveyors; any person (or organization) who promotes (advocates) the use of tests by selling testing equipment, manuals, books, or similar materials is a primary purveyor; in the case of books or articles that serve as test manuals, the primary purveyor is the author; persons who sell instruments that may be used for testing, but who do not describe or advocate specific testing procedures, are not purveyors (see **purveyor**, *secondary purveyor*, and *tertiary purveyor*)

Organization of the Standards for Primary Purveyors: Primary purveyors are obliged to provide documentation of essential elements for the tests and measurements they are promoting. Documentation should be in the form of a test manual. Most of the Standards for primary purveyors describe the elements that should be included in test manuals. Qualitative requirements for the information to be included in the manuals are presented within sections that describe what should be included in the test manuals.

P1. Persons or organizations should not become primary test purveyors unless they are prepared to adhere to the Standards.

P2. Primary purveyors of tests must provide test manuals. Books that contain major sections dealing with tests and include materials that promote and advocate the use of tests are considered test manuals, and all standards for test manuals apply to these books. Primary purveyors are responsible for the quality (accuracy) of all information in their manuals and must make every effort to ensure that information in the manuals is in compliance with the Standards (eg, research studies cited are in accordance with the Standards).

P3. Test manuals provided by primary purveyors must include descriptions of the theoretical bases of the tests and measurements, including discussions of the evidence supporting the construct validity and the content validity of the measurements. The purpose of the test must be clearly described.

P4. Test manuals provided by primary purveyors must include operational definitions.

    P4.1. Operational definitions of attributes that the test measures must be provided in the test manual.

    P.4.2. Operational definitions of terms used to describe the population for whom the test is intended must be provided in the test manual.

P.4.3. Operational definitions of terms used to describe potential test users must be provided in the test manual.

P.4.4. Operational definitions of terms used to describe components of the test or test instruments must be provided in the test manual.

P.4.5. Operational definitions of any unique terms created by the primary purveyor must be provided in the test manual.

P.4.6. Operational definitions of any terms used in a noncustomary (unusual) manner by the primary purveyor must be provided in the test manual.

P5. Test manuals provided by primary purveyors must include descriptions of the populations for whom the tests are designed. Descriptions of subjects for whom the tests should not be used and descriptions of subjects for whom the test should be used with caution must be included.

P6. Test manuals provided by primary purveyors must include descriptions of procedures that will ensure safe test administration. Safety procedures must be enumerated and should include specific instructions as to when the test should be terminated if a subject has an adverse response.

P7. Test manuals provided by primary purveyors must include descriptions of the qualifications and competencies needed by test users. These descriptions should include statements regarding potential consequences of unqualified users administering the test.

P8. Test manuals provided by primary purveyors should describe how potential test users can obtain the competencies necessary to administer the tests.

P9. Test manuals provided by primary purveyors should include narrative chronological accounts of the development of the tests, including descriptions of the development of any instruments associated with the tests.

P9.1. A description of the test developer(s) must be provided in the narrative account in the test manual.

P9.2. A description of the setting(s) in which the test was developed must be provided in the test manual.

P9.3. Documentation of the sources for any items, components, or elements used in the test must be provided in the narrative account in the test manual.

P9.4. A summary description of the history of the test, including where and how the test has been used, must be provided in the narrative account in the test manual.

P9.5. Descriptions of any revisions of the test and explanations of why revisions were made in the test must be provided in the narrative account in the test manual.

P10. Test manuals provided by primary purveyors must include descriptions of the test and associated instruments.

P10.1. Documentation of relevant technical information regarding performance characteristics of any machines, recording devices, transducers, computer interfaces, and similar instruments must be provided in the test manual.

P10.2. Descriptions of how instruments used in the test manipulate or process information in order to obtain the desired measurements must be provided in the test manual.

P11. Test manuals provided by primary purveyors must include instructions for administering the tests described in the manual. These instructions must include descriptions of all equipment and activities needed for obtaining, recording, interpreting, and reporting the measurements.

P11.1. Guidelines must be provided in the test manual as to what information and instructions should be given to the person being tested. In order to allow test users to answer questions about the test and related topics, adequate information about the test should be provided in the test manual.

P11.2. Guidelines should be provided in the test manual as to what actions persons administering the test can take to minimize the effects of extraneous factors on test performance.

P11.3. Descriptions must be provided in the test manual of the physical settings in which tests should be given and the possible effects of conducting the test in other settings.

P11.4. Descriptions must be provided in the test manual of test conditions, behaviors of persons taking the test, and other factors that could make the validity of the measurements questionable.

P11.5. Descriptions must be provided in the test manual of how the test user must manipulate or process information in order to obtain the desired measurements.

P11.6. Descriptions and instructions must be provided in the test manual for the use of any instruments required to obtain the desired measurements. This information must include, where appropriate, machine settings and any other user-selected options. The test manual must include descriptions of the effects of all options on the measurements and the consequences of selecting the incorrect options.

P11.7. If instruments are used as part of the test, the test manual must include descriptions of how the devices are calibrated. A means of testing calibration must be described in the test manual. If calibration is needed, instructions must be provided regarding a course of action to be taken.

P11.8. Descriptions must be provided in the test manual of variations in the test procedures that are available to the test user. Descriptions of variations that are known not to impair the quality of the measurements and descriptions of variations that are known to lead to measurements of questionable validity must be included.

P11.9. Background information must be provided in the test manual so that test users have the knowledge to obtain any derived measurements or categorizations necessary for interpretation of the measurements.

P11.10. Warnings must be provided in the test manual regarding the misuse of the measurements. Common errors in interpretation of the obtained measurements must be described.

P12. Test manuals provided by primary purveyors must include discussions of reactivity.

P12.1. Discussion of the degree to which administration of the test affects the measurements obtained from that test or any subsequent tests must be provided in the test manual.

P12.2. Discussion of the degree to which administration of the test may cause a change in the person taking the test must be provided in the test manual. Discussions of side effects, aftereffects and the effects of fatigue, learning, pain, and so forth may be included.

P13. Test manuals provided by primary purveyors must include evidence for all relevant forms of reliability and related information for the measurements described in the test manual.

P13.1. Descriptions of how information related to reliability was collected must be provided in the test manual, and all relevant references to peer-reviewed publications must be supplied.

P13.2. Evidence relating to reliability must be reported in the test manual in a way that describes the errors associated with common uses of the measurements.

P13.2.1 Intratester reliability estimates (indices) must be reported in the test manual. Within-day and between-day studies should have been conducted in a clinical context consistent with the intended use of the measurements. Intratester reliability should be reported in the test manual for all forms of measurements, including self-administered tests.

P13.2.2 Intertester reliability estimates (indices) must be reported in the test manual. Intertester reliability studies should have been conducted in a clinical context consistent with the intended use of the measurements.

P13.2.3 Internal consistency coefficients (or factor structures) must be reported in the test manual when there is a need to demonstrate that items or elements contributing to a measurement reflect one basic phenomenon or dimension. Studies of internal consistency should have been conducted in a clinical context consistent with the intended use of the measurements.

P13.2.4. Parallel-forms (alternative-forms) reliability must be reported in the test manual if more than one version of the test is being described. Studies of parallel-forms reliability should have been conducted in a clinical context consistent with the intended use of the measurements.

P14. Test manuals provided by primary purveyors should include descriptions of all research studies into the reliability of the measurements described in the manual, and all relevant references to peer-reviewed publications must be supplied.

P14.1. Descriptions of who conducted the reliability research must be provided in the test manual.

P14.2. Descriptions of where the reliability research was conducted must be provided in the test manual.

P14.3. Descriptions of the sample(s) studied in the reliability research must be provided in the test manual.

P14.3.1. Descriptions must be provided in the test manual of how the sample studied in the reliability research was selected.

P14.3.2. The number of subjects studied in the reliability research must be specified in the test manual.

P14.3.3. Descriptions of relevant clinical characteristics of the sample studied in the reliability research must be provided in the test manual. A discussion of how the sample is representative of the population for whom the test is intended should be included in the test manual.

P14.4. Descriptions of persons who obtained the measurements in the reliability research (ie, those who were in the role of test users) must be provided in the test manual. Descriptions of their qualifications, competencies, and experiences with the test should be included. Any special information or training given to test users prior to their obtaining the measurements in the study should be described in the test manual.

P14.5. Descriptions of the methods and research design used in the reliability studies must be provided in the test manual. The specific types of reliability that were investigated must be specified.

P14.6. Descriptions of the statistics used to derive reliability estimates and the rationale for their use must be provided in the test manual. When methodologically appropriate, reports of confidence intervals and standard errors of measurements should be included in the test manual. Examples of how the reliability estimates are to be used as part of data interpretation should be included. Reliability estimates should be accompanied by reports of regression data (ie, slopes and intercepts) when appropriate for the statistical analysis.

P15. Test manuals provided by primary purveyors must include evidence for all relevant forms of validity and related information for the measurements described in the manuals. All relevant references to peer-reviewed publications must be supplied.

P15.1. Descriptions of how information related to validity was collected must be provided in the test manual, and references to all relevant peer-reviewed publications must be supplied in the test manual.

P15.2. Evidence relating to validity must be reported in the test manual in a way that describes the errors associated with common uses of the measurements.

P15.2.1. The construct validity (theoretical basis) for the use of the measurement must be discussed in the test manual. Experimental evidence as well as logical arguments for the intended use of the measurements should be provided in the test manual.

P15.2.2. The content validity of the measurements must be discussed in the test manual. Experimental evidence as well as logical arguments for the content validity of the measurements should be provided in the test manual.

P15.2.3. Evidence for concurrent validity must be provided in the test manual when the primary purveyor contends that the measurements can be used to make inferences about the current status of an attribute at the time the measurements are obtained or shortly thereafter. This evidence must include logical and experimental data to support the use of other measurements as criteria to justify a concurrent inference. The primary purveyor should not make claims in the test manual for concurrent validity by comparing the measurement of interest with another measurement (the criterion) unless the criterion measurement has been shown to be valid (ie, it has been justified for use as a criterion).

P15.2.4. Evidence for predictive validity must be provided in the test manual when the primary purveyor contends that the measurements can be used at the time they are obtained to make inferences about the future status of an attribute. This evidence must include logical and experimental data to support the use of other measurements as criteria to justify a predictive inference. The primary purveyor should not make claims in the test manual for predictive validity by comparing the measurement of interest with another measurement (the criterion) unless the criterion measurement has been shown to be valid (ie, it has been justified for use as a criterion).

P15.2.5. Evidence for prescriptive validity must be provided in the test manual when the primary purveyor contends that the measurements can be used to determine the choice of treatment. This evidence must be based on research indicating that treatment chosen on the basis of the measurement is effective. Documentation of the effectiveness of treatment in the test manual must be based on the use of valid measurements.

P16. Test manuals provided by primary purveyors should include descriptions of all research studies into the validity of the measurements (see standard P15 for details on requirements for validity studies).

P16.1. Descriptions of who conducted the validity research must be provided in the test manual.

P16.2. Descriptions of where the validity research was conducted must be provided in the test manual.

P16.3. Descriptions of the sample(s) studied in the validity research must be provided in the test manual.

P16.3.1. Descriptions of how the sample in the validity research was selected must be provided in the test manual.

P16.3.2. The number of subjects studied in the validity research must be specified in the test manual.

P16.3.3. Descriptions of relevant clinical characteristics of the sample studied in the validity research must be provided in the test manual. A discussion should be provided in the test manual of how the sample is representative of the population for whom the test is intended.

P16.4. Descriptions of persons who obtained the measurements in the validity research (ie, those who were in the role of test users) must be provided in the test manual. Descriptions of their qualifications, competencies, and experiences with the test should be included. Any special information or training given to test users prior to their obtaining the measurements in the study should be described in the test manual.

P16.5. Descriptions of the methods and research design used in the validity studies must be provided in the test manual. The specific types of validity that were investigated must be specified in the test manual.

P16.6. Descriptions of the statistics used to derive validity estimates and the rationale for their use must be provided in the test manual. Examples of how the validity estimates are to be used as part of data interpretation should be included in the test manual. Reports of estimates of validity in the test manual should be accompanied by reports of regression data (ie, slopes and intercepts) and the standard error of the estimate when methodologically appropriate.

P17. Primary purveyors who claim that measurements can be used to classify persons into diagnostic groups based on the presence or absence of a finding (eg, cut scores or tests that result in determinations of negative or positive findings) must include in their test manuals the essential elements that allow for interpretation of these findings. In reporting these elements, the same standards as described for reports of validity must be followed.

P17.1. Percentages of false positives and false negatives must be reported in the test manual.

P17.2. Sensitivity of the test must be reported in the test manual.

P17.3. Specificity of the test must be reported in the test manual.

P17.4. Predictive values of positive and negative findings (measurements) obtained with the test must be reported in the test manual.

P18. Test manuals provided by primary purveyors must include normative data when measurements are to be interpreted in terms of how an individual measurement compares with measurements obtained on other persons (ie, when the data are norm-referenced).

P18.1. Descriptions of who obtained the normative data must be provided in the test manual.

P18.2. Descriptions of where the normative data were obtained must be provided in the test manual.

P18.3. Descriptions of the sample studied to obtain the normative data must be provided in the test manual.

P18.3.1. Descriptions must be provided in the test manual of how the sample used to obtain the normative data was selected.

P18.3.2. The number of subjects studied to obtain the normative data should be specified in the test manual.

P18.3.3. Evidence must be presented in the test manual to explain how the sample used to obtain normative data is characteristic of the population for whom the measurement is intended to be used.

P18.3.4. Descriptions of relevant clinical characteristics of the sample used to obtain the normative data must be provided in the test manual. These descriptions should include reports of the central tendencies, variabilities, and distributions of the data on relevant clinical, demographic, and anthropometric (physical) characteristics.

P18.4. Descriptions of persons who took the measurements used to obtain the normative data (ie, those who were in the role of test users) must be provided in the test manual. The test manual should include descriptions of test users' qualifications, competencies, and experiences with the test. Any special information or training given to test users prior to their taking the measurements in the study should be described in the test manual.

P18.5. Descriptions of the methods and research design used to obtain the normative data must be provided in the test manual. Normative data should be obtained using the same measurement procedures that are described in the manual. If other versions of the test were used to obtain the normative data, or if other scales were used, there must be a discussion of how the normative data relate to the data that can be obtained using the test described in the manual.

P18.6. A complete discussion of limitations in the use of the supplied normative data must be provided in the test manual. The discussion may include, but should not be limited to, considerations of whether the normative data relate to a particular local area, facility, ethnic group, age group, or gender.

P18.7. Details on any data transformations (eg, any standardization or normalization procedures) used in obtaining or preparing the normative data must be provided in the test manual.

P18.8. Primary purveyors who describe measurements that are based on interval or ratio scales should present in the test manual as part of the normative data standard scores or percentiles with accompanying measures of central tendency and variability. Data for clinically meaningful subgroups should be similarly reported in the test manual.

P18.9. Primary purveyors who describe measurements that are based on ordinal or nominal scales should present in the test manual normative data in the form of the proportion of persons in the population who can be expected to belong to each group and subgroup. Data for clinically meaningful subgroups should be similarly reported in the test manual.

P19. Test manuals provided by primary purveyors must include information that will enable a user to judge the practicality of obtaining the measurements.

P19.1. Descriptions of the number and types of personnel needed to administer the test must be provided in the test manual.

P19.2. Estimates of the time required to administer the test should be provided in the test manual.

P19.3. Descriptions of any additional equipment or supplies needed to obtain the measurements should be provided in the test manual.

P19.4. Descriptions of any potential impact on the person taking the test, in terms of the person's time and effort required and any other special requirements, should be provided in the test manual.

P19.5. Descriptions of any potential risks or hazards, and means for reducing the risks and hazards, to persons taking the test of administering the test must be provided in the test manual.

P20. Test manuals provided by primary purveyors must include discussions of any special considerations concerning the test and resulting measurements. For example, subgroups for whom measurements may be invalid should be identified, as should persons for whom a test may represent some psychological or physical risk.

P21. Test manuals provided by primary purveyors must include descriptions of all special groups for whom the test is contraindicated or known to lead to measurements of questionable validity.

P22. Test manuals provided by primary purveyors must include descriptions of a mechanism by which test users can communicate with the primary purveyor regarding the test. The mechanism should allow the user to seek further information, share observations and results, or report problems.

P23. Test manuals provided by primary purveyors must include a bibliography that provides references specific to the test and pertinent to the content of the test. The bibliography must be organized in such a manner that references supporting the scientific basis for the test are differentiated from references dealing tangentially with the test or simply reporting that the test has been used.

P24. A primary purveyor's promotional material for a test or measurement must not make claims that exceed what can be justified by existing research. When information about a test or measurement is provided in promotional material, that material should meet the same standards of accuracy and freedom from misleading impressions that apply to the test manual (this standard is based on that found in the *Standards for Educational and Psychological Tests*: American Psychological Association, Washington, DC, 1974, page 10). Any primary purveyor who chooses to discuss the tests or measurements of another purveyor in promotional materials should do so only while maintaining the same standards of accuracy and freedom for misleading impressions that apply to the test manual.

P25. Primary purveyors should make every reasonable effort to notify test users and potential users of any modifications or revisions in tests or test manuals.

P26. Primary purveyors who administer tests as part of test development must make every reasonable effort to observe the Standards for Test Users.

Standards for Secondary Test Purveyors (indicated with an S)

The Standards in this section describe requirements for secondary purveyors of tests. The following is the definition of a secondary purveyor.

Secondary purveyor: any researcher or other person who publishes a scholarly work that examines aspects of tests and who, in that scholarly work, suggests (advocates) that a test be used; a secondary purveyor is not the initial source of information on a test (ie, did not supply the manual or the original information on the test) (see **purveyor**, *primary purveyor*, and **tertiary purveyor**)

Organization of the Standards for Secondary Purveyors: Secondary purveyors may have limitations imposed upon them regarding the information they can supply in published reports. The Standards have been written in a way that takes into account these limitations. However, the Standards do list the elements that should be included in written materials prepared by secondary purveyors. Using the Standards as a guide, secondary purveyors may, when publication limitations are too stringent, have to decide whether the integrity of their reports may be excessively compromised by the requirements for publication. Secondary purveyors are obligated to reconsider whether, in the face of such limitations, they choose to remain secondary purveyors.

S1. Persons or organizations should not become secondary test purveyors (ie, advocates of using tests) unless they are prepared to adhere to the Standards. A scholarly publication that describes tests or uses of tests does not make an author a test purveyor unless advocacy of specific test use is part of that publication. Care should be taken in such publications to differentiate analysis, research, and discussion from advocacy.

S2. Secondary purveyors who advocate the use of tests or measurements must be prepared to support that advocacy. In journal articles, the advocacy should not exceed what can be supported through documentation. Secondary purveyors, therefore, should be aware of the limitations imposed by journals publishing their reports. Secondary purveyors who publish in other forums or who are not presenting a research report should attempt to supply more information than can be expected in a typical published research report.

S3. Secondary purveyors must include in all their research reports or scholarly papers the basic elements that will ensure credibility. Secondary purveyors should make every reasonable effort to publish their reports in peer-reviewed journals, which ordinarily require the basic elements for credibility.

S4. Secondary purveyors must include in all of their research reports or scholarly papers sufficient detail to allow for replication of their research.

S5. Secondary purveyors must include descriptions of the theoretical bases for the test and measurements they discuss in research reports or scholarly papers. A discussion of the evidence relating to the construct validity and the content validity of the measurements should be included. The purpose of the test must be clearly described. The length of these discussions should be to the extent allowed in the publication in which the report will or may appear.

S6. Secondary purveyors should include, to the extent allowed in the publication in which their report will or may appear, operational definitions related to all aspects of the tests and measurements they discuss.

    S6.1. Operational definitions of attributes that the test measures must be provided in reports by secondary purveyors.

    S6.2. Operational definitions must be provided for terms used to describe the population for whom the test is intended in reports by secondary purveyors.

    S6.3. Operational definitions of terms used to describe potential test users must be provided in reports by secondary purveyors.

    S6.4. Operational definitions of terms used to describe components of the test or test instruments must be provided in reports by secondary purveyors.

    S6.5. Operational definitions of any unique terms created by the secondary purveyor must be provided in reports by secondary purveyors.

    S6.6. Operational definitions of any terms used in a noncustomary (unusual) manner by the secondary purveyor must be provided in reports by secondary purveyors.

S7. Research reports or scholarly papers written by secondary purveyors must include, to the extent allowed in the publication in which the report will or may appear, a description of the population for whom the test is designed. Descriptions, based on research of the secondary purveyor, of subjects for whom the test should not be used and descriptions of subjects for whom the test should be used with caution should be included.

S8. Research reports or scholarly papers written by secondary purveyors should include, to the extent allowed in the publication in which the report will or may appear, descriptions of the qualifications and competencies of persons who use (administer) the tests being discussed.

S9. Research reports or scholarly papers written by secondary purveyors should include, to the extent allowed in the publication in which the report will or may appear, a brief account of the development of the test being discussed.

S10. Research reports or scholarly papers written by secondary purveyors must include, to the extent allowed in the publication in which the report will or may appear, a description of the test being discussed and associated instruments.

    S10.1. Documentation of relevant technical information regarding performance characteristics of any machines, recording devices, transducers, computer interfaces, and similar instruments must be provided in reports by secondary purveyors. Regardless of whether this information is published, a secondary purveyor must, upon request, be prepared to provide this information by personal communication.

    S10.2. Research reports or scholarly papers written by secondary purveyors must include descriptions of how instruments manipulate or process information in order to obtain the measurements being discussed.

S11. Research reports or scholarly papers written by secondary purveyors must include instructions for conducting the test being discussed. These instructions must include, to the extent allowed in the publication in which the report will or may appear, descriptions of all activities needed for obtaining measurements, for recording measurements, and for interpreting measurements. Regardless of whether this information is published, a secondary purveyor must, upon request, be prepared to provide this information by personal communication.

    S11.1. Research reports or scholarly papers written by secondary purveyors should include guidelines on the information that is to be given to the persons being tested. These guidelines should include the instructions given to the persons being tested.

    S11.2. Research reports or scholarly papers written by secondary purveyors should include descriptions of the physical settings in which the test should be given and the possible effects of conducting the test in other settings.

    S11.3. Research reports or scholarly papers written by secondary purveyors should include descriptions of test conditions, behaviors of persons taking the test, and other factors that could make the validity of the measurements questionable.

    S11.4. Research reports or scholarly papers written by secondary purveyors should include descriptions of how the data were manipulated or processed in order to obtain the measurement being discussed.

    S11.5. Research reports of scholarly papers written by secondary purveyors should include descriptions and instructions of how instruments were used to obtain the measurements being discussed. This information must include, where appropriate, machine settings and any other user-selected options. A discussion of the possible effects of any option on the measurements and the consequences of selecting the incorrect options should be included.

S11.6. Secondary purveyors who describe the use of instruments in their reports should include descriptions of how the instruments used to obtain the measurements are calibrated.

S11.7. Research reports or scholarly papers written by secondary purveyors should include sufficient background information so that readers can understand how any derived measurements or categorizations were made, especially if this information is necessary for interpretation of the measurements.

S11.8. Research reports or scholarly papers written by secondary purveyors must include warnings regarding misuse of the measurements being discussed. If research indicates that common errors in interpretation of test data can occur, secondary purveyors must describe these errors in their reports.

S12. Research reports or scholarly papers written by secondary purveyors should include, to the extent allowed in the publication in which the report will or may appear, discussions of special considerations concerning the test and measurements being discussed.

S12.1. Secondary purveyors should include discussions of reactivity in their reports.

S12.1.1. Research reports or scholarly papers written by secondary purveyors should include discussions of the degree to which administration of the test being discussed affects the measurement obtained from that test or any subsequent tests.

S12.1.2. Research reports or scholarly papers written by secondary purveyors should include discussions of the degree to which administration of the test being discussed may cause a change in the person taking the test. Discussions of side effects, aftereffects, and the effects of fatigue, learning, pain, and so forth may be included.

S13. Secondary purveyors who author research reports or scholarly papers that examine reliability must include in those reports, to the extent allowed in the publication in which the report will or may appear, essential elements that would allow for interpretation of the report.

S13.1. Research reports or scholarly papers on reliability written by secondary purveyors should include a thorough and critical review of what is known about the reliability and the validity of the measurements being discussed.

S13.2. Research reports or scholarly papers on reliability written by secondary purveyors must include a detailed description of the sample studied.

S13.2.1. Research reports or scholarly papers on reliability written by secondary purveyors must include descriptions of how the sample studied in the reliability research was selected.

S13.2.2. Research reports or scholarly papers on reliability written by secondary purveyors must specify the number of subjects studied.

S13.2.3. Research reports or scholarly papers on reliability written by secondary purveyors must include descriptions of relevant clinical characteristics of the sample studied. A discussion of how the sample is representative of the population for whom the test is intended should be provided by the secondary purveyor.

S13.3. Research reports or scholarly papers written by secondary purveyors must include descriptions of persons who obtained the measurements in reliability studies (ie, those who were in the role of test users). Descriptions of the test users' qualifications, competencies, and experiences with the test should be included. Information or special training given to test users prior to their obtaining the measurements in the study should be described by the secondary purveyor.

S13.4. Research reports on reliability written by secondary purveyors must include descriptions of the methods and research designs used in their studies. The specific types of reliability being investigated must be specified.

S13.5. Research reports on reliability written by secondary purveyors must include a description of the statistics used to derive reliability estimates. The rationale for the use of these statistics must be provided. When methodologically appropriate, reports of confidence intervals and standard errors of measurement should be included. Examples of how the reliability estimates are to be used as part of data interpretation should be included. A reliability estimate should be accompanied by a report of regression data (ie, slopes and intercepts) when appropriate for the statistical analysis.

S14. Secondary purveyors who author research reports or scholarly papers that examine validity must include in those reports, to the extent allowed in the publication in which the report will or may appear, elements that allow for interpretation of the report.

S14.1. Research reports or scholarly papers on validity written by secondary purveyors should include a thorough and critical review of what is known about the reliability and the validity of the measurements being discussed.

S14.2. Research reports on validity written by secondary purveyors must include descriptions of the methods and research designs used in their studies. The specific types of validity investigated must be specified by the secondary purveyor. Descriptions of the sample(s) studied in the validity research must be provided. These descriptions should include the number of subjects studied and how these subjects were selected.

S14.3. Research reports or scholarly papers written by secondary purveyors must include evidence of validity to support each inferential use of the measurement suggested by the secondary purveyor. The design must be appropriate to support arguments of the presence of each relevant type of validity.

S14.4. Research reports on validity written by secondary purveyors must include descriptions of the statistics used to derive validity estimates. The rationale for the use of these statistics must be provided. When methodologically appropriate, reports of confidence intervals and standard errors of the estimate should be included. Examples of how the validity estimates are to be used as part of data interpretation should be included. Validity estimates should be accompanied by reports of regression data (ie, slopes and intercepts) when appropriate for the statistical analysis.

S14.5. Secondary purveyors who state in research reports or scholarly papers that measurements can be used to make inferences about the current status of an attribute at the time the measurements are obtained or shortly thereafter must include logical and experimental data to support the use of other measurements as criteria to justify these concurrent inferences. Secondary purveyors should not make claims for concurrent validity by comparing the measurement of interest with another measurement (the criterion) unless the criterion measurement has been shown to be valid (ie, it has been justified for use as a criterion).

S14.6. Secondary purveyors who state in research reports or scholarly papers that measurements can be used at the time they are obtained to make inferences about the future status of an attribute must include logical and experimental data to support the use of other measurements as criteria to justify these predictive inferences. Secondary purveyors should not make claims for predictive validity by comparing the measurement of interest with another measurement (the criterion) unless the criterion measurement has been shown to be valid (ie, it has been justified for use as a criterion).

S14.7. Secondary purveyors who state in research reports or scholarly papers that measurements can be used to determine the choice of treatment (ie, prescriptive validity) must base these statements on research indicating that treatment chosen on the basis of the measurement is effective. Documentation of the effectiveness of treatment must be based on the use of valid measurements and should be included in reports by the secondary purveyors.

S15. Secondary purveyors who claim in research reports on scholarly papers that measurements can be used to classify persons into diagnostic groups based on the presence or absence of a finding (eg, cut scores or tests that result in determinations of negative or positive findings) must report the essential elements that allow for interpretation of these findings. In reporting these elements, the same standards as described for reports of validity must be followed. This information should be supplied to the extent allowed in the publication in which the report will or may appear.

S15.1. Percentages of false positives and false negatives must be described in reports by secondary purveyors.

S15.2. Sensitivity of the test must be described in reports by secondary purveyors.

S15.3. Specificity of the test must be described in reports by secondary purveyors.

S15.4. Predictive values of positive and negative findings (measurements) obtained with the test must be described in reports by secondary purveyors.

S16. Secondary purveyors who include normative data in their reports must include, to the extent allowed in the publication in which the report will or may appear, essential elements required for the interpretation of these normative data.

S16.1. Secondary purveyors must describe who (ie, the researcher) obtained the normative data they report.

S16.2. Secondary purveyors must describe in their reports where the normative data were obtained.

S16.3. Secondary purveyors must describe in their reports the sample studied to obtain the normative data.

S16.3.1. Secondary purveyors must describe in their reports how the sample used to obtain the normative data was selected.

S16.3.2. Secondary purveyors must specify in their reports the number of subjects studied to obtain the normative data.

S16.3.3. Secondary purveyors must explain in their reports how the sample used to obtain the normative data is characteristic of the population for whom the measurement is intended to be used.

S16.3.4. Secondary purveyors must describe in their reports relevant clinical characteristics of the sample used to obtain the normative data. These descriptions should include reports of the central tendencies, variabilities, and distributions of the data on relevant clinical, demographic, and anthropometric (physical) characteristics.

S16.4. Secondary purveyors must describe in their reports the persons who took the measurements used to obtain the normative data (ie, those who were in the role of test users). Descriptions of test users' qualifications, competencies, and experiences with the test should be included. Any special information or training given to test users prior to their obtaining the measurements in the study should be described by the secondary purveyor.

S16.5. Secondary purveyors must describe in their reports the methods and research designs used to obtain the normative data. Normative data should be obtained using the same measurement procedures that are described in the report. If other versions of the test were used to obtain the normative data, or if other scales were used, there must be a discussion of how the normative data relate to the data that can be obtained using the test described in the report.

S16.6. Secondary purveyors must supply in their reports a complete discussion of limitations in the use of the normative data they report. The discussion may include, but should not be limited to, considerations of whether the normative data relate to a particular local area, facility, ethnic group, age group, or gender.

S16.7. Secondary purveyors must supply in their reports details on any data transformations (eg, any standardization or normalization procedures) used in obtaining and preparing the normative data they are reporting.

S16.8. Secondary purveyors who report normative data for measurements that are based on interval or ratio scales should present as part of the normative data standard scores or percentiles with accompanying measures of central tendency and variability. Data for clinically meaningful subgroups should be similarly reported.

S16.9. Secondary purveyors who report normative data for measurements that are based on ordinal or nominal scales should present the normative data in the form of the proportion of persons in the population who can be expected to belong to each group and subgroup. Data for clinically meaningful subgroups should be similarly reported.

S17. Advocacy by secondary purveyors for the use of a measurement must not exceed a level that can be supported by the research of the secondary purveyor or by other published data.

Standards for Tertiary Test Purveyors (indicated with a T)

The Standards in this section describe requirements for tertiary purveyors of tests. The following is the definition of a tertiary purveyor.

Tertiary purveyor: any person who teaches or prepares instructional material that describes specific tests or specific uses of measurements; this definition includes, but is not limited to, persons teaching in academic institutions, clinical educators, and continuing educators who are not acting in the role of primary or secondary purveyors (see **purveyor**, *primary purveyor*, and *secondary purveyor*)

Organization of the Standards for Tertiary Purveyors: Tertiary purveyors have two primary obligations: to understand tests and measurements in general and to have specific knowledge about the tests they discuss. The first part of these Standards describes general knowledge that a tertiary purveyor should have, and many of the subsequent Standards describe what information a tertiary purveyor should supply for each test the tertiary purveyor discusses. Tertiary purveyors, because they interact with potential test users, must be prepared to provide additional information to these potential users upon request. Some of the Standards describe the type of information that a tertiary purveyor should be prepared to supply during discussions.

T1. Persons should not become tertiary purveyors unless they are prepared to adhere to the Standards and unless they understand the requirements for primary and secondary purveyors. Persons should also not become tertiary purveyors unless they understand the requirements for test users and are willing to assist potential test users in complying with those Standards.

T2. Tertiary purveyors must have a basic knowledge of the theory and principles of tests and measurements.

    T2.1. Tertiary purveyors must understand what constitutes a measurement, what constitutes a test, and the role of instruments in obtaining measurements.

    T2.2. Tertiary purveyors must understand the differences between clinical opinions (impressions) that are not based on valid measurements and inferences that are based on the use of valid measurements.

    T2.3. Tertiary purveyors must understand what constitutes an operational definition and the importance of using operational definitions.

    T2.4. Tertiary purveyors must understand the different levels of measurement (ie, nominal, ordinal, interval, and ratio) and the mathematical operations that are appropriate for each level.

    T2.5. Tertiary purveyors must understand types of reliability and validity and how these qualities relate to clinical decisions and other uses of measurements.

    T2.6. Tertiary purveyors must understand the methods used to assess reliability and validity (eg, statistics and research designs).

    T2.7. Tertiary purveyors must understand the relationship between reliability and validity and the differences between the two qualities.

    T2.8. Tertiary purveyors must understand what constitutes meaningful normative data and how such data can be used.

T2.9. Tertiary purveyors must understand the differences between objective measurements and subjective measurements and the implications of using each type of measurement.

T2.10. Tertiary purveyors must understand the meaning and use of the terms "false negatives," "false positives," "true negatives," "true positives," "predictive value of a measurement," "specificity of a test,"and "sensitivity of a test."

T2.11. Tertiary purveyors must understand the importance of knowing the technical specifications of instruments.

T2.12. Tertiary purveyors must understand the importance of calibrating instruments.

T2.13. Tertiary purveyors must understand the methods and effects of normalizing or standardizing measurements.

T2.14. Tertiary purveyors must understand the meaning and implications of reactivity to tests.

T3. Tertiary purveyors should promulgate the Standards for Test Users and, in their teaching, should provide potential test users with the necessary tools and information so that these potential test users can adhere to user standards.

T4. Tertiary purveyors, when discussing a test, must provide descriptions of the theoretical bases for the test and must discuss evidence relating to construct and content validity.

T5. Tertiary purveyors must provide all relevant operational definitions during their discussions of a test.

T5.1. Tertiary purveyors must provide operational definitions for attributes that the test measures.

T5.2. Tertiary purveyors must provide operational definitions for terms used to describe the population for whom the test is intended.

T5.3. Tertiary purveyors must provide operational definitions for terms used to describe potential test users.

T5.4. Tertiary purveyors must provide operational definitions for terms used to describe components of the test or test instrument.

T5.5. Tertiary purveyors must provide operational definitions for any terms created by purveyors.

T5.6. Tertiary purveyors must provide operational definitions for any terms they use in a noncustomary manner.

T5.7. Tertiary purveyors must provide operational definitions for any terms they modified or created.

T6. Tertiary purveyors, during discussions of a test, must provide a description of the population for which the test is designed. Descriptions of subjects for whom the test should not be used and descriptions of subjects for whom the test should be used with caution should be included.

T7. Tertiary purveyors have an obligation to review critically what is known about the reliability and validity of tests that they discuss, including how statistics were used to assess reliability and validity. Tertiary purveyors must also be prepared to answer questions of potential test users regarding reliability and validity studies and statistics used in these studies.

T8. Tertiary purveyors must provide all information that is available when they convey or discuss normative data.

T8.1. Tertiary purveyors must describe the methods used to obtain the sample that was used to obtain the normative data. The generalizability of the normative data must be characterized relative to the sampling method.

T8.2. Tertiary purveyors must describe the sample studied (eg, the number of subjects and the distributions of relevant clinical, demographic, and anthropometric [physical] characteristics). How this group is characteristic of the population for whom the test is intended must also be discussed.

T8.3. Tertiary purveyors must discuss limitations in the normative data. This discussion may include, but should not be limited to, considerations of whether the data relate to one local area, facility, ethnic group, age group, or gender.

T8.4. Tertiary purveyors must discuss details on any data transformations used and whether any standardization or normalization procedures were used in generating the normative data.

T8.5. Tertiary purveyors who discuss measurements that are interval or ratio scaled must provide standard scores or percentiles with measurements of central tendency and variability, if these data are available. Data for meaningful subgroups should be similarly reported. If these data are lacking, the tertiary purveyor should discuss the limitations in the use of the normative data.

T8.6. Tertiary purveyors who discuss measurements that are ordinal or nominal scaled or who describe classifications must provide normative data in terms of the proportion of persons in the population that can be expected to belong to each group, if this information is available. Data for meaningful subgroups should be similarly reported. If these data are lacking, the tertiary purveyor should discuss the limitations in the use of the normative data.

T9. Tertiary purveyors, in discussing a specific test, must provide descriptions of the qualifications and competencies needed by the test user to administer that test.

T10. Tertiary purveyors, when discussing a specific test, should provide a brief account of the development of the test.

T11. Tertiary purveyors, in discussing a specific test, must provide descriptions of the test and instruments associated with the test.

T11.1. Tertiary purveyors must discuss available documentation of relevant technical information regarding performance characteristics of any machines, recording devices, transducers, computer interfaces, and similar instruments. The tertiary purveyor should identify the source of this documentation. If documentation is not available, the tertiary purveyor must discuss the implications and limitations of using such instruments.

T11.2. Tertiary purveyors must describe how instruments used in the test manipulate or process information in order to obtain the measurements, if this information is available. Tertiary purveyors should identify the source of this information. If this information is not available, the tertiary purveyor must discuss the implications and limitations of using such instruments.

T12. Tertiary purveyors must provide instructions for administering all tests that they teach to potential test users. These instructions must include descriptions of the sources for test manuals as well as all equipment and activities needed for obtaining, recording, and interpreting the measurements.

T12.1. Tertiary purveyors must provide guidelines for what information and instructions are to be given to the person being tested. Information about the test should be provided that will allow the potential test user to answer questions about the test and related subjects.

T12.2. Tertiary purveyors must describe the physical settings in which the test should be given and possible effects of conducting the test in other settings.

T12.3. Tertiary purveyors must describe conditions, behaviors of persons taking the test, or other factors that could make the validity of the measurements questionable.

T12.4. Tertiary purveyors must describe how the test user must manipulate or process information in order to obtain the desired measurements.

T12.5. Tertiary purveyors must provide instructions to potential test users for use of any instruments required to obtain the desired measurements. These instructions, where appropriate, must include machine settings and any other user-selected options. Descriptions of the effects of all options on the measurements and the consequences of selecting the incorrect options should be included.

T12.6. Tertiary purveyors who discuss tests that involve the use of instruments must describe how the instruments are calibrated. A means of testing calibration must be described. If calibration is needed, the tertiary purveyor must provide instructions regarding a course of action to be taken.

T12.7. Tertiary purveyors must describe variations in the test procedures that are available to the test user. Descriptions of variations that are known not to impair the quality of the measurements and descriptions of variations that are known to lead to measurements of questionable validity must be included.

T12.8. Tertiary purveyors must provide background information so that potential test users will have the knowledge to obtain any derived measurements or categorization necessary for interpretation of the measurements.

T13. Tertiary purveyors must provide warnings regarding misuse of the measurements they discuss. Common errors in interpretation of the measurements must be described. If research or the tertiary purveyor's experience indicates that errors in interpretation of test data can occur, then these errors should be described.

T14. Tertiary purveyors must discuss the implications of reactivity when discussing a test.

T14.1. Tertiary purveyors must discuss the degree to which administration of the test affects the measurement obtained from that test or any subsequent tests.

T14.2. Tertiary purveyors must discuss the degree to which administration of the test may cause a change in the person taking the test. Discussions of side effects, after-effects, fatigue, learning, and so forth may be included.

T15. Tertiary purveyors must include in their discussions of a test descriptions of all special groups for whom the test is contraindicated or known to lead to measurements of questionable validity.

T16. Tertiary purveyors, when discussing measurements used to classify persons into groups based on the presence or absence of a diagnostic finding (eg, use of cut scores or tests to determine a positive or negative finding), must discuss the limitations of these measurements.

    T16.1. Tertiary purveyors must report the percentages of false positives and false negatives for the measurements they discuss. If this information is not available, tertiary purveyors must discuss the limitations of using these measurements.

    T16.2. Tertiary purveyors must report the sensitivity of the tests they discuss. If this information is not available, tertiary purveyors must discuss the limitations of using these tests.

    T16.3. Tertiary purveyors must report the specificity of the tests they discuss. If this information is not available, tertiary purveyors must discuss the limitations of using these tests.

    T16.4. Tertiary purveyors must report the predictive values of positive and negative findings for the measurements they discuss. If this information is not available, tertiary purveyors must discuss the limitations of using these measurements.

T17. Tertiary purveyors, when they discuss a test, must identify any way in which their versions of the test differ from published versions of the test. Tertiary purveyors must also discuss how these variations can affect the measurement and the uses of the measurement. A tertiary purveyor who modifies a test becomes a primary purveyor and must meet the Standards specified for primary purveyors.

T18. Tertiary purveyors must provide information that will enable potential test users to understand the limitations of tests that do not meet the Standards. Tertiary purveyors must take potential test users aware of the limited justifiable inferences that can be made from tests that do not meet the Standards.

T19. Tertiary purveyors must discuss with potential test users issues related to the interpretation of the measurements they discuss. Tertiary purveyors must warn potential test users of common errors that the purveyors know occur in clinical practice. Strategies for avoiding these errors should be discussed.

T20. Tertiary purveyors must discuss with potential test users how results of tests must be reported. Tertiary purveyors must discuss what information is essential in reports.

T21. Tertiary purveyors must discuss with potential test users the difference between clinical opinions and interpretations that are based solely on valid measurements. The tertiary purveyor must also provide examples of how clinical opinions may be differentiated from test findings in clinical reports and other communications.

T22. Tertiary purveyors must assist potential test users in understanding the role of specific measurements in the clinical decision-making process. Tertiary purveyors must characterize whether existing research justifies conclusions based on single tests or whether clinical decisions should be the result of the synthesis of multiple measurements.

Standards for Test Users (indicated with a U)

The Standards in this section describe requirements for test users. The following is the definition of a test user.

Test user: one who chooses tests, interprets test scores, or makes decisions based on test scores (this definition is from *Standards for Educational and Psychological Tests.* American Psychological Association, Washington, DC, 1974, page 1)

Organization of the Standards for Test Users: Four basic types of Standards are found in the Standards for Test Users. The Standards listed first detail the general knowledge that a test user must have. The majority of the Standards in this section deal with specific requirements that a user should consider when performing specific tests. These Standards include issues relating to the choice of tests, the performance of testing, observing the rights of test takers, and the use of obtained measurements. The last two Standards, U44 and U45, describe the requirements test users should observe in interpreting and reporting test results.

U1.   Persons should not become test users unless they are prepared to adhere to the Standards and understand the requirements for test purveyors.

U2.   Test users must have a basic understanding of local, state, and federal laws governing the use of tests in their practice settings.

U3.   Test users must have a basic knowledge of the theory and principles of tests and measurements.

> **U3.1.**   Test users must understand what constitutes a measurement, what constitutes a test, and the role of instruments in obtaining measurements.

> **U3.2.**   Test users must understand the differences between clinical opinions (impressions) that are not based on valid measurements and inferences that are based on the use of valid measurements.

> **U3.3.**   Test users must understand what constitutes an operational definition and the importance of using operational definitions.

> **U3.4.**   Test users must understand the different levels of measurement (ie, nominal, ordinal, interval, and ratio) and the mathematical operations that are appropriate for each level.

> **U3.5.**   Test users must understand types of validity and how these types of validity relate to the use of measurements.

> **U3.6.**   Test users must understand types of reliability and validity and how these qualities relate to clinical decisions and other uses of measurements.

> **U3.7.**   Test users must have a basic understanding of the methods used to assess reliability and validity (eg, statistics and research designs).

> **U3.8.**   Test users must understand the relationship between reliability and validity and the differences between the two qualities.

> **U3.9.**   Test users must understand what constitutes meaningful normative data and how such data can be used.

U3.10. Test users must understand the differences between objective measurements and subjective measurements and the implications of using each type of measurement.

U3.11. Test users must understand the meaning and use of the terms "false negatives," "false positives," "true negatives," "true positives," "predictive value of a measurement," "specificity of a test," and "sensitivity of a test."

U3.12. Test users must understand the importance of knowing the technical specifications of instruments.

U3.13. Test users must understand the importance of calibrating instruments.

U3.14. Test users must have a basic understanding of the methods and effects of normalizing or standardizing measurements.

U3.15. Test users must understand the meaning and implications of reactivity to tests.

U4. Test users must have background knowledge in basic, applied, and clinical sciences related to the selection, administration, and interpretation of each test they use.

U5. Test users must understand the theoretical bases (construct and content validity) for the tests they use, and they must have knowledge about the attribute (characteristic) being measured.

U6. Test users must be familiar with the development of tests that they use and the test settings in which those tests have been developed and used.

U7. Test users must understand how a test they are using relates to similar tests or previous versions of the same test.

U8. Test users must be able to justify the selection of tests they use. Test users must also be prepared to supply logical arguments to justify the rejection of tests they choose not to use.

U8.1. Test users must consider the safety of subjects in selecting tests and should consider the benefits to be obtained from a test in view of potential risks to the subject.

U8.2. Test users should consider the practicality of the test (eg, personnel, time, equipment, cost of administration, and impact on the person taking the test) in selecting tests and in planning examination procedures.

U9. Test users must be able to identify their sources of information regarding tests they use. Test users must be able to specify where they obtained information (eg, rationale and directions) for selecting and conducting a test.

U9.1. Test users should not cite a test manual as a source of information unless they have personally examined a complete copy of the test manual. Test users should not conduct tests unless they have examined all relevant sections of a complete copy of the test manual.

U10. Test users must understand all operational definitions related to tests they use.

U10.1. Test users must understand the operational definitions for attributes that the test measures.

U10.2. Test users must understand the operational definitions for terms used to describe the population for whom the test is intended.

U10.3. Test users must understand the operational definitions for terms to describe potential test users.

U10.4. Test users must understand the operational definitions for terms used to describe components of the test or test instruments.

U10.5. Test users must understand the operational definitions for any terms created by purveyors of the test.

U10.6. Test users must be able to identify and understand the operational definitions for any terms used in a noncustomary matter.

U11. Test users must be able to describe the population for whom the test was designed. Test users must be able to relate this description to the persons they are testing.

U12. Test users must be able to determine before they use a test whether they have the ability to administer that test. The determination should be based on an understanding of the test user's own skills and knowledge (competency) as compared with the competencies described by the test purveyor.

U12.1. Test users must be able to describe the potential consequences of administering a test that they do not have the skills or knowledge to administer.

U12.2. Test users who have doubts about their ability to administer a test should report this information when they report test results (eg, their reservations about the quality of their measurements should be discussed).

U13. Test users must follow instructions provided by purveyors for all tests they administer.

U13.1. Test users must understand instructions for administering all tests that they use. Test users must be able to describe all of the equipment and activities needed for obtaining, recording, and interpreting the measurements. Test users must be able to identify the source of the instructions.

U13.2. Test users who deviate from accepted directions for obtaining a measurement should not use published data or documentation relative to reliability and validity to justify their use of the measurement.

U14. Test users must know what information and instructions are to be given to the person being tested. Test users should be able to answer questions about the test and related subjects.

U14.1 Test users who do not give the purveyor's specified instructions to persons being tested, or test users who are unable to give these instructions, should not use published data or documentation relative to reliability and validity to justify their use of the measurements.

U15. Test users must know the physical settings in which the test should be given and the possible effects of conducting the test in other settings.

U16. Test users must be able to identify any conditions or behaviors in the person being tested that may compromise the reliability or validity of their measurements (eg, if a modified position must be used in manual muscle testing because of a deformity). Test users who observe such conditions or behaviors should note these observations in their reports of any resultant measurements. Test users who believe that the effect on their measurements could be significant should include a discussion of the implications of these observations in their reports.

U17. Test users must have a basic understanding of the instruments they use as part of a test.

    U17.1. Test users must know relevant technical information regarding performance characteristics of any machines, recording devices, transducers, computer interfaces, and similar instruments they use. Test users should be able to identify the source of this information. If this information is not available, the test user must be able to discuss the implications and limitations of using such instruments.

    U17.2. Test users must be able to describe how instruments they use manipulate or process information in order to obtain measurements. Test users should identify the source of this information. If this information is not available, the test user must be able to discuss the implications and limitations of using such instruments.

U18. Test users must know how to use any instruments required to obtain the desired measurements. This Standard includes, where appropriate, the test user knowing how to choose machine settings and other user-selected options. Test users must be able to discuss the effects of all options on their measurements and the consequences of selecting the incorrect options.

U19. Test users must be able to describe how instruments they use for a test are calibrated, including the means of testing calibration. Tests users must know the course of action to be taken when calibration is needed.

U20. Test users, for all the tests they use, should be able to describe variations in the test procedures that are available. Test users must be able to describe variations that are known not to impair the quality of the measurements and those variations that are known to lead to measurements of questionable validity.

U21. Test users who deviate from accepted directions for obtaining a measurement should not use published data or documentation relative to reliability and validity to justify their use of the measurement.

    U21.1. Test users who administer tests in settings other than those recommended by the purveyor should not use published data or documentation relative to reliability and validity to justify their use of the measurement.

U22. Test users have a responsibility to suggest further testing when they have serious concerns about the quality of the measurements they obtain or when they believe that other tests or other personnel can be used to obtain better measurements.

U23. Test users who are required to derive or transform measurements must have sufficient training and knowledge to derive or transform those measurements. Test users must have the background information and skills needed to derive measurements or make categorizations necessary for interpretation of their measurements (eg, how to normalize or standardize a score or how to classify a measurement).

U24. Test users must be aware of any normative data for the measurements they are obtaining (see Standard U44.3 for guidelines on using normative data to interpret measurements; see Standard U45.10 for guidelines on reporting measurements related to normative data). Test users should be able to evaluate critically normative data and use the data for clinical decision making.

U25. Test users must make every effort to control the environment (test setting) in which they test in order to maintain consistent conditions between tests. These efforts are needed to ensure that the validity and reliability of a measurement are not compromised.

U26. Test users must make every effort when personal information is being obtained to control the environment (test setting) in which they administer tests in order to preserve the privacy of the person taking the test.

U27. Test users must be able to discuss common errors in the interpretation of the measurements they use.

U28. Test users must make every effort to minimize the effects of reactivity associated with the tests they use.

U29. Test users should report to the purveyor of the test any problems regarding a test or any associated instruments.

U30. Test users should communicate with other test users and purveyors regarding their experiences with tests.

U31. Test users must avoid getting persons prior knowledge about the nature of a test when such knowledge is known to compromise the validity of the measurements.

U32. Test users are responsible for maintaining confidentiality of test results. Confidentiality of results should be in accordance with standard practices in the institution or community in which the test user obtains the measurements. Results should not be shared with any persons (or organizations) who are known to be unwilling to respect the right of confidentiality of the person who was tested.

U33. Test users should not share results of tests with persons (or organizations) who are likely to misuse that information.

U34. Test users must respect the rights of persons whom they test.

    U34.1. Test users must respect the right of persons to refuse to be tested. Test users must allow persons to discontinue participation in any test at any time without recrimination or prejudice against that person.

    U34.2. Test users must inform persons whom they test of potential risks and benefits that persons may experience as a result of taking the test.

    U34.3. Test users must respect the right of persons being tested to know the results of tests, the interpretations of those test results, and with whom the test results will be shared. The right of the person to know the results of tests does not imply that all test users must personally supply this information. In some cases, test results may be supplied by the professional who originated a referral or who is coordinating treatment.

    U34.4. Test users who fail to adhere to the Standards and who use tests inappropriately, especially in terms of drawing unwarranted conclusions from results, violate the rights of persons being tested.

        U34.4.1. Test users who misrepresent their clinical opinions as being based on test results when evidence for such opinions is not found in the research literature violate the rights of persons taking tests. (For example: A test user may use a battery of tests to determine the ability of a patient with low back pain to function in an industrial environment. In this hypothetical example, the test battery yields a measurement that is supposed to predict the type of work that the patient may do safely. There is, in this example, evidence for the validity of this inference. However, based on the test user's observations, the test user concludes that the patient is malingering. This is the test user's clinical opinion; it is not based on the validated use of the measurement. The test user does not violate the rights of the person taking the test by having or presenting clinical opinions, but would violate the person's rights by contending that the measurement could be used to infer malingering.)

U35. Test users must maintain records in such a manner that information about tests and measurements is accurate and is not likely to be distorted or lost. Abbreviations used in communications should be limited to those that appear in established references.

U36. Test users have a responsibility to report inappropriate test use to proper authorities.

U36.1. Test users who know that a person's rights are not being observed during testing must make every effort to change that situation.

U37. Test users should select tests based on what is best for the person being tested. Test selection based on considerations of personal benefit to the test user, test purveyor, or the referring practitioner is inappropriate.

U38. Test users, in clinical practice, should avoid the use of tests that were designed solely for research purposes. Such tests, when they are used in the clinical setting, should be identified in all reports as research tests that have not necessarily been shown to be reliable or valid in clinical use.

U39. Test users should not assign persons to conduct tests unless they know that such persons are qualified to conduct the tests.

U40. Test users should not make promotional claims for their testing procedures that are not supported by research literature.

U40.1. Test users are responsible for the critical evaluation of all claims of test purveyors and should not merely repeat the claims of purveyors without critical evaluation of these claims.

U41. Test users should assist in the development and refinement of testing procedures by sharing their knowledge of tests and assisting in the collection of data where appropriate.

U42. Test users have a responsibility to periodically review the test procedures they and their colleagues use in their institutions (practice settings) to ensure that appropriate use of measurements is being made and that the rights of persons tested are being observed.

U42.1. Test users, as part of their periodic review of test procedures, should examine whether the normative data they are using appear to relate to their clinical setting.

U42.2. Test users, as part of their periodic review of test procedures, should attempt to estimate the reliability of measurements in their practice settings. All forms of reliability relevant to the practice settings should be assessed.

U43. Test users who use tests that do not meet the Standards should be aware that these tests do not meet the Standards. Test users, therefore, should interpret results of these tests with caution and share these reservations with all persons who receive test results.

U44. Test users must follow the basic rules and principles of measurement when they interpret results of tests they use. (The following Standards provide guidelines for interpreting measurements. These Standards are not meant to supersede or in any way modify the requirements specified elsewhere in the Standards for Test Users.)

U44.1. Test users must limit their interpretations of measurements to the inferences for which those measurements have been shown to be valid.

U44.2. Test users must consider the error associated with their measurements when they interpret their test results. Reliability and validity estimates should be considered when the test user makes interpretations of measurements. (For example: Reliability studies have indicated that a measurement varies as much as 10% between repeated tests. Therefore, a change of less than 10% on that measurement may be due, at least in part, to measurement error. Test users who note changes the second time they take measurements should consider, before they make interpretations, that the change may not reflect real change, but may be due solely to measurement error.)

U44.3. Test users must consider whether normative data are available for the measurements they interpret. Test users must consider the sources of the normative data and how applicable these data are to the measurements they are interpreting.

U44.3.1. Test users should use all available information when using normative data for interpretations of measurements.

U44.3.1.1. Test users using normative data should interpret any measurement that is interval or ratio scaled in terms of how that measurement relates to measures of central tendency, measures of variability, and percentiles.

U44.3.1.2. Test users using normative data should interpret any measurement that is nominal or ordinal scaled in terms of the proportion of persons in the population that can be expected to belong to the same classification.

U44.4. Test users must consider the limitations of their measurements when they classify persons into diagnostic groups based on the presence or absence of a finding (eg, use of cut scores or tests to determine a positive or negative finding). Test users should use all available data in making their interpretations.

U44.4.1. Test users must consider the percentages of false positives and false negatives for a diagnostic test when interpreting measurements. If this information is not available, test users should understand the limitations of making interpretations based on their measurements.

U44.4.2. Test users must consider the sensitivity of the diagnostic test they are using when they interpret their measurements. If this information is not available, test users should understand the limitations of making interpretations based on their measurements.

U44.4.3. Test users must consider the specificity of the diagnostic test they are using when they interpret their measurements. If this information is not available, test users should understand the limitations of making interpretations based on their measurements.

U44.4.4. Test users consider the predictive values of positive and negative findings when they interpret their measurements obtained with a diagnostic test. If this information is not available, test users should understand the limitations of making interpretations based on their measurements.

U44.5. Test users must avoid overinterpreting the results of their tests. Test users are responsible for understanding both the certainty and the uncertainty with which they can make judgments based on their measurements.

U44.6. Test users must consider whether changes (eg, attributable to development or learning) in the person being tested may alter performance on subsequent tests. Test users, when appropriate, should discuss in their reports of test results the possibility of change in the future. Test users should not imply that a test result represents an immutable state when there is reason to believe that the test result may differ if the test is repeated at some future time.

U44.7. Test users must consider the conditions under which they conduct tests and the extent to which results are generalizable to other test situations (eg, testing in other places or at other times).

U44.8. Test users must identify whether their interpretations are based on the results of multiple measurements obtained with the same test or on the results of a single measurement.

U44.9. Test users must identify whether any of their interpretations are not supported by research evidence of validity. Such interpretations must be clearly identified as being based on the test user's personal opinion.

U45. Test users reporting the results of tests must supply adequate information so that these results can be understood. (The following Standards provide guidelines for reporting about measurements. These Standards are not meant to supersede or in any way modify the requirements specified elsewhere in the Standards for Test Users.)

U45.1. Test users should specify, when more than one form of a test exists, the specific form of the test used when they report their results.

U45.2. Test users should report measurements in the form specified by the purveyor's instructions. Test users should justify any deviations from standard methods of reporting.

U45.3. Test users should use only the terms that are defined in test manuals or in other supporting literature when they discuss tests or measurements. Descriptive terms that are not defined should be avoided, because such terms may encourage inappropriate interpretation of results.

U45.4. Test users, in reporting test results, should use terms in a customary manner or describe how terms are being used differently. Test users should justify deviations from commonly accepted uses of terms in their reports.

U45.5. Test users must consider estimates of reliability and validity when reporting test results. Test users should report estimates of the errors associated with a measurement when they report test results. (For example: Reliability studies have indicated that a measurement varies as much as 10% between repeated measurements. Therefore, a change of less than 10% may be due, at least in part, to measurement error. Test users who note changes the second time they take measurements, in reporting such measurements, should also report that the change in the measurement may not reflect real change. The change may be solely due to measurement error. A report of the reliability estimate or standard error, in this case, would be useful in the test user's report.)

U45.6. Test users should include warnings about common misinterpretations of their measurements in reports of their measurements.

U45.7. Test users should report any significant effects of reactivity when they report the results of their tests.

U45.8. Test users who use a variation of a test must indicate, when they report test results, that a variation was used. The test users must note whether they believe that the variation may have affected the quality of their measurements. Test users who believe the variation had a significant effect on the measurements should discuss this belief in all reports of test results.

U45.9. Test users should report any aspect of the test that may cast doubt on test results (eg, ways in which the person tested differed from the population for which the test was designed or any observation the test user made during testing).

U45.10. Test users, in reports of test results, should relate their measurements to normative data, if available. Test users should report the source of the normative data they use and, if necessary, discuss how applicable the data are to the measurements they are reporting (see Standard U44.3 for guidelines on using normative data to interpret measurements).

U45.10.1. Test users using normative data, when they report test results, should report all information necessary to understand the test user's interpretation of the measurements.

U45.10.1.1. Test users using normative data for measurements that are interval or ratio scaled should report their test results in terms of how the measurements relate to measures of central tendency, measures of variability, and percentiles.

U45.10.1.2. Test users who report classifications in their test results should also report the proportion of persons in the population who can be expected to belong to that classification. The test user, if requested, should be able to cite the source of the data used to determine the proportions.

U45.11. Test users reporting the results of their tests should indicate whether any data were transformed (normalized or standardized). Test users, in their reports, should justify the use of transformations, if this is not customary practice.

U45.12. Test users who base their interpretations of test results on the mean of multiple measurements should note this fact in their reports of test results. Test users should justify the use of the mean of multiple measurements in clinical reports, if this is not customary practice.

U45.13. Test users who base their interpretations on a single measurement chosen from a group of measurements (eg, the best of three trials) should note this fact when they report test results. Test users, in their reports, should justify the use of the single measurement and the criteria used to select the measurement, if this is not customary practice.

U45.14. Test users who base their interpretations on the results of a variety of tests should note this fact when they discuss their measurements. Test users should justify their selection of the tests in reporting test results.

U45.15. Test users should note in their reports of test results the specific criteria they use for clinical decisions. When a specific measurement (eg, cut score) is used for a clinical decision, the test user, in all reports, should justify the use of that specific measurement.

Standards for Ensuring Integrity in Measurement Research
(Indicated with an R)†

R1. Physical therapists who conduct measurement research should maximize the integrity of their work by following the guidelines set forth in the Standards for Tests and Measurements sections on primary and secondary purveyors.‡

R2. Physical therapists must ensure that subjects in measurement studies are volunteers and that no coercion or deception was used to entice subjects to volunteer. Participation of each volunteer should be based on the subject's (or the subject's legally authorized representative's) understanding of the nature of the study and its expected risks and benefits.

R2.1. Physical therapists who conduct measurement research must obtain, in writing, informed consent from subjects or the subjects' legal representatives before the subjects participate in studies. The form of the consent must be in accord with appropriate laws, regulations, and institutional requirements.

R2.2. Physical therapists who conduct measurement research must assure their subjects or the subjects' legal representatives, in writing, of the subjects' right to withdraw consent and discontinue participation in the measurement study. Such participation in the measurement study. Such withdrawal should not result in any prejudice against or negative impact upon the subject.

R2.3. Physical therapists who obtain informed consent as part of measurement research must inform their subjects of the subjects' legal representatives, in writing, of the extent to which confidentiality will be maintained.

R3. Physical therapists must ensure that information about subjects obtained during measurement research is recorded, stored, and reported in ways that protect the subjects' right to confidentiality.

---

† The *Standards* are adapted from the document *Integrity in Physical Therapy Research*, which was approved by the APTA Board of Directors in March 1985 and modified in November 1987.

‡ The *Standards for Ensuring Integrity in Measurement Research* describe specific requirements that should be met by researchers. Researchers may be primary or secondary test purveyors and will, almost always, be test users; therefore, researchers must comply with all relevant Standards described in those sections.

R3.1. Physical therapists who conduct measurement research, before they use any information about the subjects, must inform their subjects or the subjects' legal representatives about this planned action. The subjects or the subjects' legally authorized representatives must authorize, in writing, the release of this information. This information includes any data or recorded images of the subjects.

R4. Physical therapists who conduct measurement research are expected to ensure the privacy of subjects during the course of their measurement research. Therapists, if more than one subject must be present during a test session, should ensure that each subject has the maximum possible privacy.

R5. Physical therapists who conduct measurement research must minimize the risk of physical, psychological, or social harm to their subjects.

R6. Physical therapists who conduct measurement research must be guided at all times by a concern for the physical, psychological, and social well-being of their subjects.

R7. Physical therapists who use patients as subjects during measurement research must comply with the applicable laws regulating the practice of physical therapy in the jurisdiction in which the study is taking place.

R8. Physical therapists must make every effort to comply with the requirements governing the approval and conduct of measurement research within the institutional or organizational setting in which they conduct research. If the setting has no requirements governing the approval of proposals for measurement studies, physical therapists should assist in developing and implementing such requirements.

R9. Physical therapists who seek institutional approval and external funding for measurement research must provide accurate information to institutional review boards, funding agencies, and other relevant groups.

R10. Physical therapists who conduct measurement research that has been approved by an institutional review board or a funding agency are obligated to adhere to the approved protocol and to deviate from that protocol only in accordance with the policies of the board or agency that granted approval.

R11. Physical therapists who conduct measurement research must ensure that reports of their studies are accurate and represent only the work that was done in the study.

R12. Physical therapists must conduct measurement research in such a way that the prospect of financial gain or past financial assistance to the investigators or their institutions has no influence on the results or the manner in which the results are reported.

R12.1. Physical therapists must report all sources of financial support for a study when the results of their study are published.

R13. Physical therapists must make every effort to share information about their measurement studies and findings in an appropriate manner.

R13.1. Physical therapists should submit formal research reports to journals in which the manuscript will be subjected to meaningful peer review.

R13.2. Physical therapists should honor the requests of professional colleagues for access to their measurement research data.

R14. Physical therapists must have a thorough knowledge of measurement theory and pertinent professional and scientific literature before they conduct measurement studies. Measurement studies must be carried out with due consideration given to this body of knowledge.

R15. Physical therapists who conduct measurement research are obligated to know their personal limitations and to know when to seek consultation and peer review of their research plans before they begin data collection.

R16. Physical therapists, in written reports of measurement studies, must ensure that all references are correct and that citations are used appropriately. References must directly support information in the sentence in which the references are cited. If the references supply indirect support for the statement, this support should be indicated.

R17. Physical therapists must describe, in written reports of measurement studies, all relevant information in adequate detail so that readers may replicate the study.

R18. Physical therapists must describe, in written reports of measurement studies, steps that were taken to comply with governmental and institutional regulations governing research in the setting in which the study was carried out. The report should include descriptions of the steps that were taken to ensure subjects' rights.

R19. Physical therapists who are participating in measurement studies must dissociate themselves from any activities that are unethical or unlawful. Physical therapists must make every effort to take corrective action when they encounter unethical, unlawful, or incompetent acts in the conduct of measurement research. In addition, they are obligated to report any unethical, unlawful, or incompetent acts of any person to the appropriate authorities.

R20. Physical therapists must assist the profession in documenting the integrity of measurement research. Physical therapists called upon to assist in inquiries about any measurement research should cooperate. There should be no recriminations against any person called upon to serve as an investigator. A person should not investigate any other person's work unless that person possesses the necessary knowledge and skills to evaluate objectively all available data.

Index